PSORIASIS:
THE STRUGGLE AND THE TRIUMPH

A Healthy Transformation for Everyone Living with Psoriasis

Elliott Douglas Derzaph

© 2003 by Elliott Douglas Derzaph. All rights reserved.

No part of this book may be reproduced, stored in a retrieval system, or transmitted by any means, electronic, mechanical, photocopying, recording, or otherwise, without written permission from the author.

ISBN: 1-4107-0216-2 (Paperback)

Library of Congress Control Number: 2003090038

This book is printed on acid free paper.

Printed in the United States of America
Bloomington, IN

ATTENTION ORGANIZATIONS & BUSINESSES

This book supplied by the Publisher is available at quantity discounts with bulk purchases for educational use, business or sales promotion or for fund raising. Special books or book excerpts can also be created to fit specific needs. For details contact the Publisher at the address above.

PRINTED IN THE UNITED STATES OF AMERICA

Includes bibliographical references.

1. Psoriasis - Popular works.
2. Psoriasis - Alternate treatment
3. Psoriasis - Self-help.
4. Psoriasis - Health
5. Title.

1stBooks – rev. 07/18/03

What Others Are Saying About This Book

[This book] encompasses a very diverse study of the many alternative treatments for this chronic condition."

Linda A. Henley
National Secretary, The Psoriasis Association
Northampton, England

A wonderful book. Diverse, personal and timely. A healthy key thread throughout the book is understanding our emotions and the need to manage our excesses.

Over the years, many subjects have crossed my desk but little has been made available to the public on the topic of psoriasis. My medical experience recommends this book as an essential tool, that will encourage doctor and patient to work together as a healing team. It will also help the people living with the psoriasis sufferers to understand this unique disease.

Psoriasis: The Struggle and The Triumph is a wealth of information, a handbook. It generates insights to the abundant resources hidden just below the surface. Further, it stresses the importance of nutrition, exercise and a healthy, emotional stress-free attitude. Mr. Derzaph's book gives us the key to the sane interaction of Psoriasis sufferers and non-sufferers.

Velma Scott, M.D., D.C., Ph. D.
Texas

I am amazed at the amount of research that Mr. Derzaph has accomplished. As an experienced Registered Nurse I have been in constant touch with the author over a number of years. I have recommended some of the author's treatments to psoriasis patients and am happy to say that many of them have been better able to cope. Many people with psoriasis, or those with friends and families who have this condition, will benefit greatly from this book. I know they will be greatly helped, emotionally and physically, and will be better able to cope with the stress this condition creates.

Nullis Mohammed, R.N.
New York

"*Psoriasis: The Struggle and The Triumph*" will be beneficial to all those with psoriasis who wish to take an active role in their health care. In fact, the author advocates such a stance. After 17 years of research, Mr. Derzaph has assembled in one place, most, if not all, the methods and techniques for ameliorating or healing this stubborn condition.

In a most helpful way, Mr. Derzaph presents external methods from nature and from conventional medicine, as well as, non-toxic, internal, natural healing procedures. All of his sources are well documented and numerous resources are provided in the text.

Most interesting of all, is the author's experience with the mind-emotion-body connection, which I have observed, as a clinician, is an often hidden, but essential, key to the healing process. As he tells his own story, Elliott Derzaph encourages the reader to bring this key to the conscious level of awareness, rather than depend upon random luck for healing. His clarity and courage to present this material is both timely and ground breaking for psoriasis sufferers everywhere.

I recommend this book to members of the general public, patients and their caregivers, and to all professionals involved in the treatment of psoriasis.

Fred Siciliano, O.M.D., L.Ac., MM.
California

Dedication

To my beautiful, loving wife, Wendy, who, through her love and support, encouraged me to write this book and who spent countless hours proofreading the manuscript.

And

To my mother, Virginia, for sharing her love, history, and suggestions.

And

To my son, Ethan, for his love of life.

Notice

The information contained in this book is prepared from sources that are believed to be accurate and reliable. Readers are advised to seek the advice and assistance of their personal health care professional(s) before proceeding with any new health care program or making changes in any existing health care program.

There is nearly always disagreement among medical professionals regarding the effectiveness of treatment regimens for psoriasis. The resulting conflicting medical recommendations underscore the need - indeed, the absolute necessity - of every patient becoming **personally responsible** for his/her own treatment. With only rare exception, should the doctor be looked to as an oracle from which issues "true knowledge," rather than as a resource for guidance and consultation.

Guidelines

You must accept the reality of psoriasis. You must be the one in control, if you aren't, then the psoriasis governs your life. It is always your choice who runs the show.

It is well documented that even a minor amount of psoriasis symptoms cause great negative affects to our quality of life including restricting public activities, lack of self-confidence, depression and intimacy with others.

You must become less passive; less like an object to be taken in a shopping bag to the doctor.

While it is widely accepted that emotional management is the key to dealing successfully with a patient's disease, most doctors do not address this point.

Take in all the information you can find, adapt it to your own situation, and use each part to help solve your problem.

It is important to feel and express how psoriasis influences you.

It is vital to find comfort for yourself and your family when you are in public view or engaging in any type of social interaction.

When you have taken back full responsibility for yourself, you can then find others who will be willing to help you.

My hope is that each person reading this book will gain at least one new insight into improving his/her ability to live with psoriasis and experience a full rich life.

Sharing Your Own Story

Elliott Douglas Derzaph, the author of this book, has done a most remarkable job in assembling seventeen years of study and research into the book you are about to read.

But the author is fully aware that the study of diseases is a dynamic process, and new discoveries can be made on almost a daily basis.

In addition, psoriasis is a unique disease - in that much of the research is done by the sufferers, rather than solely by medical researchers. Therefore, the author knows that the publication of this book is likely to bring hundreds of individuals "out of the woodwork," to describe treatments that might be known only to themselves.

Thus, Mr. Derzaph, the author, invites all readers to do the following:

First, to share any information you believe would be useful to other psoriasis sufferers, so that it might be assembled into a form suitable for dissemination. You may either send an email to - "Info@PsoriasisAdvisor.com" or send a note to - Psoriasis Advisor, P.O. Box 643038, West Los Angeles, CA 90064-3038.

Second, if you wish to regularly receive new information, please contact a national psoriasis organization in your country (addresses in the Appendix) they can provide us with the best coverage.

Foreword

As a psychiatrist in active practice, I frequently see the physical and psychological suffering that occurs when individuals must manage a chronic illness, like psoriasis, day after day. It's amazing how often they say, no one has ever really explained it to me - which greatly adds to the fear and helplessness! Elliott Derzaph has addressed this problem for psoriasis sufferers, with the kind of empathy and compassion that only comes from having experienced the disorder himself.

His book is encyclopedic in scope, but still entirely readable for the average person. It covers up-to-the-minute medical research about psoriasis, while still focusing on practical approaches to achieve relief now. We may have to wait another decade for the gene(s) responsible for this disorder to be identified and the defective functioning permanently reversed, but until then this book fills a much-needed role for every psoriasis sufferer.

Melissa Derfler, M.D., Ph. D.
Diplomate, American Board of Psychiatry and Neurology

Acknowledgments

I owe my thanks to hundreds of people who offered advice and information in the preparation of this book.

A few friends and associates offered particularly valued contributions. I extend my sincerest thanks to these people:

    Ken Abel - Editor
    Sherith Decker – Executive Liaison of N.P.F.
    Wendy Derzaph - Wife & Attorney
    Dr. Melissa Derfler - Psychiatrist
    Clair Gold, H.W., M. - Counselor
    Nullis Mohammed - Registered Nurse
    Virginia Pinel - My Mother
    Dr. Velma Scott - Acupuncturist
    Dr. Fred Siciliano - Acupuncturist
    Palisades Advertising & Marketing
    Institute of Advanced Thinking
    WEE Research & Marketing

Three organizations that helped me the most in dealing with psoriasis were:

    Ontological Learning Center of the Pacific
    The National Psoriasis Foundation and
    The Psoriasis Society of Canada

The doors, these organizations opened in my mind allowed me to look beyond my doctors' paths and proved to be a godsend.

The value of the information that these organizations can supply cannot be overstated. To help support their activities I have become a member of all three.

The Ontological and Emotional Intelligence education taught to me, throughout my early adulthood, was significant to the point of redirecting my whole life.

I tithe 10% of the proceeds from this book because of my respect and admiration for the goals and achievements of Ontology and Emotional Intelligence.

These organizations are referred to, frequently, within the text. Further explanation of the work of these organizations will be found in the Appendix. Applications for membership for the organizations are also included. I highly recommend contributions to non-profit organizations.

Contents

Dedication v

Notice vii

Guidelines ix

Sharing Your Own Story... xi

Foreword xiii

Acknowledgments xv

Introduction 1

Chapter 1
Insights to Psoriasis: The Basic Facts........................ 8

Chapter 2
Putting out the Burn: Topical Solutions & Treatments...... 12

Chapter 3
Letting the Sun Shine In: Exposure to Sunshine or Light........ 21

Chapter 4
Refreshed by Water: The Benefits of H2O 25

Chapter 5
Savoring your Life: Massage...................................... 27

Chapter 6
The Last Resort: Surgery 30

Chapter 7
Caring for Hair, Nails and Ears.................................. 33

Chapter 8
How to Dress functionally with Psoriasis................. 35

Chapter 9
Physical Activity benefits your overall Health as well as helping to control Psoriatic Arthritis 37

Chapter 10
What your Body's Organs can be telling You or just things to Know 41

Chapter 11
Unleashing the Natural Physician Inside: Acupuncture and Chiropractic 49

Chapter 12
New and Traditional Medications/Drugs 59

Chapter 13
European Remedy: GH3? 62

Chapter 14
Nutrition Health Options 64

Chapter 15
The Natural Approach: Vitamins, Minerals and Herbs 71

Chapter 16
Fasting: Clearing the Mind and Body without Starving 79

Chapter 17
A Healthy Colon: Internal Washing Cleanses the Body 83

Chapter 18
Mind and Body together again: Mental Exercises 86

Chapter 19
Healing Imagery: Seeing Yourself Clearly 90

Chapter 20
Freeing Dis-Ease: The Path To Emotional Intelligence® 93

Chapter 21
A Personal Journey 102

Chapter 22
Conclusions: Evolution of Our Hopes... 106

Chapters Digest 109

Appendices 119

Glossary 121

Optimum Schedule & Curriculum 127

Education 129

Psoriasis Information Resources And Organizations Throughout The World 130

References & Product Resources 135

Home Therapy Lighting 140

Memebership Information and Applications 142

A Poem 151

About the Author 153

Psoriasis: The Struggle and the Triumph
A Healthy Transformation for Everyone Living with Psoriasis

Introduction

There are millions of people who currently live with Psoriasis: specifically eight million Americans and Canadians; one and a half million in the United Kingdom and Ireland; and sixty to eighty million other people on this planet. In the United States, Psoriasis affects one person in fifty with 200,000 new cases diagnosed each year of which 20,000 are children. Disability benefits are granted to several hundred people with debilitating psoriasis. In the United States between two and three percent of the population have Psoriasis. In Canada, Psoriasis affects one in 33 people. Crohn's, arthritis, and diabetes are often diseases associated with Psoriasis. Crohn's disease is seven times more likely to develop in people with Psoriasis. Psoriasis, for unknown reasons, responds to many different types of treatments.

This Psoriasis guide for everyone living with Psoriasis is about awareness, education, daily living, treatment options and possible cures for this temporarily "incurable" disease. This book will save you money, assist you in achieving greater comfort in life, and aid you in enjoying better health. Until a cure is found, I hope to provide various processes of healing. Psoriasis is a controllable disease that can last your life time.

I became afflicted with psoriasis in 1978 and have successfully managed the disease since 1993. From the time of onset to the present, I have been gathering information about the disease and its treatments, from family, friends and associates; from others afflicted with the disease; from doctors and medical journals; and from psoriasis research organizations throughout the world. The observations and conclusions resulting from over twenty years of interactions are presented in this book.

Psoriasis: The Struggle and The Triumph covers as complete a spectrum of treatments as is known at the time of publication. I share with you my personal insights along with documented medical research. Treatments range from the standard medical approaches to lesser known - even obscure - choices. My goal is to provide those afflicted with psoriasis with the best and most up-to-date and uncensored information available.

I want to satisfy the thirst for information that most psoriasis patients have after they are first diagnosed. And I want to help the "veterans" of psoriasis who wish to be made aware of the latest treatments. Most of all, I would like to offer hope by presenting new choices and alternatives.

Psoriasis patients assume that their source of medical care is the most informed; or, at the very least, is attuned to new possibilities for care or cure. Unfortunately, the reality is that most medical professionals simply can't keep up with all the changes and diversity of choices, while, simultaneously, handling their existing workload. Keep in mind that there are a few hundred products to treat Psoriasis in the marketplace at anytime.

The vast majority of patients have no idea that there are numerous, easily accessible resources, rich in therapeutic possibilities, which are unknown to the majority of medical practitioners.

Psoriasis: The Struggle and The Triumph presents a multitude of such therapies, which are mostly simple, natural and non-medical in nature, and which can be used to augment, even the best, professional medical care.

No other book, describing psoriasis therapies and available in the English speaking countries of the world, contains more than a fraction of the information provided in this book.

As both a guide to other resources, and as a resource in itself, *Psoriasis: The Struggle and The Triumph* offers psoriasis patients new topics for discussion with their doctors. It is vital that the patient be well informed and knowledgeable about health choices so that the patient and doctor, working together, can make the best possible decisions.

During the last twenty plus years I have watched people endure pain because they were not aware of the huge body of knowledge which could have helped reduce or eliminate their pain. I have also seen numerous patients, myself included, waste thousands of dollars on treatments that didn't work. (Some years ago, I spent well over 8 weeks of income on a two week program at a health institute, for treatment that resulted in only a minor physical change.)

Here are some of the reasons that serious problems can result if you, as a psoriasis sufferer, take no responsibility for your own treatment; and instead, put yourself totally in the hands of your doctor.

- Doctors frequently do not address their patients' emotions even though it is widely acknowledged that emotional management is key to dealing successfully with the disease.

- Doctors are taught how to help you, when you are sick, rather than, how to help you maintain good health.

- Doctors make mistakes and, at times, may not be willing to admit them. Being informed helps you identify those mistakes.

- Doctors are very busy. Few doctors are able to keep up with the changes, latest discoveries and developments in the treatment of diseases (other than those that are their particular interest or specialty) or take the time to make a patient feel cared for.

- Doctors, drug companies and the American Medical Association (A.M.A.) are in the business of treating people who are ill; and they promote the profitability of the medical industry.

- Doctors are part of their own herd consciousness: it is safer to "follow the pack."

- Doctors often have difficulty acknowledging non-medical complementary treatment regimens such as nutrition, stress management and chiropractic.

Participation, rather than the cold, observational stance served up by many doctors, is what is needed. Doctors should spend more personal time with their patients so they may be really in touch.

A psychoanalyst, who was a good friend of mine, told me many times that when he started out as a doctor it was so different than it is today. He said the change in attitude, especially, in his exchange with doctors, took a toll on him. Often doctors, upon discovering he was also a doctor, would completely change the subject being discussed and ask, "So what are you invested in?" and other such financial commentary, and, rarely returned to any discussion on standard medical topics let alone the latest greatest medical discoveries.

It is important to know the limitations of the people who advise us or who work with us in treating our disease. But, it is invaluable for us to know how we can help ourselves. The goals we choose will direct us to the best ways to rid ourselves of psoriasis. The idea is not to blame or devalue the medical world's capabilities... but to see the value of looking beyond its limitations.

We make an incorrect assumption if we believe that someone else is willing to be totally responsible for our health. This book was written to show there are more effective alternatives for those willing to help themselves. Work with your health care professionals while becoming as knowledgeable as possible about all aspects of psoriasis care. Be responsible for your own health and recognize that "when you feel good about who and what you are, you can greatly speed the healing process." Recently, the term mind-body approach has been used to describe the activity of assisting in your own health care.

I have collected information on psoriasis from books, magazines, newspapers, newsletters, and numerous personal conversations. I have discussed psoriasis with people from the United States, Canada, Mexico, Central America, the Middle East, Great Britain, Europe and Eastern Europe. I have been filling my bookcases and files with information for years. Through the encouragement of my wife, Wendy, I decided to write this book to share the knowledge I accumulated. My hope is that each person reading this book will gain at least one new insight, allowing his/her to improve his/her ability to live with psoriasis.

I have spent untold thousands of dollars in attempts to help myself. I spent several thousand dollars one year trying yet another "totally new" cure, hoping that this time the psoriasis would go away for a few months or maybe longer. At the same time, I was praying for it to leave for years. Sometimes, my most fervent wish or prayer was to not see a plaque again for the rest of my life.

Just as each person's appearance is individually unique, so too is his/her body chemistry. Furthermore, since the effectiveness of treatments for psoriasis seems to depend, in part, on body chemistry, each treatment may have a different effect on different individuals.

Many approaches are available for psoriasis treatment, each having its own benefits and drawbacks. This book was written to help you choose or design your health program. Take in all the information you can find, adapt it to your own situation and use the parts that help solve your problem. I spent many years gathering information on psoriasis treatments in hopes of opening new paths of discovery, so that new successes with psoriasis, including a cure, might come about. As more information is made available to a more diverse audience, we create a larger pool of individuals who can use this information to seek and find solutions.

What follows is a Psoriasis Bill of Rights propounded by the National Psoriasis Foundation (N.P.F.). My suggested additions and/or modifications are included, in parentheses.

1. You have the right to the most potent treatment that will give the best results with the mildest (or no) side effects.

2. You have the right to a full explanation of psoriasis and any treatments or medications that are prescribed.

3. You have the right to sympathetic (empathetic), courteous treatment from your physician (health care practitioner).

4. You have the right to change doctors or pharmacies; to ask for a second opinion; and to comparison shop for good buys in prescription and over-the-counter products.

5. You have the right to be angry, depressed, or upset because you have psoriasis. (And the right to learn processes to release each of these negative emotions so that your energy may be used constructively.)

6. You have the right to ask for support and encouragement from family members (and friends).

7. You have the right to learn all you can about psoriasis and its treatment.

8. You have the right to tell others that you have psoriasis and to describe it from a medical and scientific point of view.

9. You have the right (emotionally and physically) to deal with psoriasis in your own way and on your own terms, and not as other people think you should.

10. You have the right to see yourself as a person (with self-belief) and of great worth who has a diagnosed medical condition - psoriasis.

(From "Psoriasis Bill of Rights," an N.P.F. Bulletin, copyright 1984. Reprinted by permission of National Psoriasis Foundation.)

Dian Dincin Buchman, wrote the following in her book, Herbal Medicine:

> Recent studies indicate that people who feel helpless may contract a serious chronic disease as a result, and sometimes do not recover their health precisely because they perceive themselves as totally helpless.
> Thus, life-saving technology produced a more dependent, less self sufficient person. Old health concepts based on simple and useful observations vanished. People were ashamed to talk about

the value of sunshine; about walking outdoors to feel better; about how the "best two doctors" are the right and left foot; about breathing deeply to eliminate stress, "sweating it out,"; about spring cures (body cleansing after long, hard winters). Rough, chewy, "old fashioned" food was rejected, and devitalized white bread, as delicious as library paste, took its place along with soft foods, hormone-injected meat, and chemicalized fruits and vegetables. Alas, the number of chemicals added to food is so large, that it is said a Thanksgiving meal will provide a thousand chemicals. My friend, Beatrice Trum Hunter, describes this state of events as "the great nutrition robbery."

Although people are living longer, they are not necessarily feeling better, and there has been a vast interest in exercise programs, water as therapy, and drugless home doctoring. People are rediscovering their strong ethnic roots and reinvestigating old values.

You must try to become less passive, less like an "object" to be taken in a shopping bag to the doctor. And some people do think of themselves as a sort of a package they can deposit on the doctor's desk: "Here, Doc, take this, and see what you can do" - almost the way you take a radio or a car in to be fixed.

A holistic approach means you will not list only the symptoms, but you will try to unearth the causes of the symptoms. Sometimes the cause will be obvious, and you can immediately alleviate or eliminate the causal factors. Other times, reasons for a symptom will be hidden, but since you will be thinking about it, an idea may pop out to redirect your activities. Be a detective. It's amazing how many problems you can solve for yourself. But if the headache persists, see a physician in any case.

(From Herbal Medicine, by Dian Dincin Buchman, Gramercy 1980 edition, copyright 1979 by Random House, Inc. Reprinted by permission.)

While reading the January 12, 1992 Parade magazine supplement to my local newspaper, I came upon an article written by Gloria Steinem. One sentence grabbed my attention because of my discomfort with psoriasis: Ms. Steinem said, "I've also realized that focusing on parts of my body that I like - and trying to imagine expanding that feeling to the rest of me - is a key to the whole-body pride that should be everyone's birthright."

I think it is most important to learn to "live" with psoriasis. The collection and understanding of information on psoriasis clarifies your health goal and reduces the anxiety, while you work to reduce or remove psoriasis in your life. The body maintenance you must perform because of your psoriasis should become just as much a part of your daily routine as brushing your teeth and showering.

Personal experience is the best teacher and it is the only way to fully understand what psoriasis is all about. Frank, a corporate executive and longtime friend, told me that despite watching me go through broken bones, bad relationships, career changes and other personal losses, nothing compared to the pain and the challenge I went through with psoriasis.

I wrote this book with the intention of presenting a complete and informative guide which could help ease the pain of the millions living with psoriasis. Perhaps my most significant discovery was the role played by emotions and stress. For example, the stress caused by difficult economic times causes many psoriasis patients to suffer flare-ups. This causes further emotional upset, which in turn causes more stress. The effect of emotions and stress is taken up in detail in this book.

"The Heartbreak of Psoriasis," is a commercial phrase, annoying to most psoriasis sufferers. But it is an all revealing statement just the same. I cannot suggest that by reading this book your psoriasis will disappear. I can, however, state that by being well informed so that you can help yourself, you will play a major part in relieving the ache of living with your psoriasis. It is my hope that this book will help turn "heartbreak" into "happiness" for many readers.

Elliott Douglas Derzaph

1 Insights to Psoriasis: The Basic Facts

My first experience with doctors specializing in psoriasis was at U.C.L.A. Medical Center. After noticing what I thought was a rash, I made an appointment to visit the Dermatology Department. The doctor who attended to me made a few quick notes and then disappeared for a couple of minutes. With my approval, he returned to the room with five interns in tow to observe me as I sat in my underwear. He then had the interns gather around and pointed at the plaques, exclaiming, *"Here you can see a classic case of psoriasis."* From the very beginning, I wasn't thrilled to be a "classic case."

A sample psoriasis patient has five things in common with millions of others who have psoriasis:

1) Psoriasis is different because each case is unique.

2) What works for some might not work for you.

3) What works for you might not work for others.

4) A treatment may work well once, not as well the second time, and then not at all.

5) You don't know why you have it.

The most peculiar, yet common, remarks about psoriasis that come up in discussions are *"no solution seems to work straight across the board,"* and/or *"what works for me won't work for others."* The only blanket solutions are general health measures such as good eating habits. Also, maintaining good emotional health, **especially with regard to self-belief and stress management**, is a major factor. Having patience and not expecting quick results can be a tremendous aid in keeping the disease in check.

Psoriasis appears to be a misfiring of the body's immune response. Psoriasis is an immunologic disorder that appears as a condition of the skin that affects about three percent of the population of the U.S.A. and Canada. Psoriasis is not contagious and can be brought under temporary control with the proper medical treatment. For most individuals, the disease's biggest discomfort is its appearance, second only to the continual itching. Psoriasis is relatively harmless, and is reversible.

Psoriasis is hereditary and will frequently skip a generation. Psoriasis patients can usually name other members of their family who have had the disorder. Family members inherit the psoriasis mutant gene and develop psoriasis; or they can be carriers, passing it on to their children without developing the disease themselves. (The heredity factor had caused me - great pain and regret - to refrain for many years from having children of my own.)

It appears that specific factors cause inception in each individual. Infections can initiate psoriasis. Stress, in forty percent of psoriasis sufferers can, not only bring on psoriasis for the first time, but can also be responsible for a relapse. It is very important to understand that if you are anxious or under pressure you increase the likelihood of being predisposed to psoriasis. Therefore, you should attempt to understand and control stress and anxiety, two factors which are also important determinants in your overall health.

A friend of mine sent me a photocopy of a chapter from a book (title unknown), written by a physician. The chapter's title was: "The Skin you Live In: Psoriasis Need Be No Heartbreak." On the final page the author stated: *"Acquire a philosophical attitude toward life's problems. Don't let other people get under your skin."*

Exposure to sunlight can be very beneficial in the treatment of the disease; however, if overdone, resulting in sunburn, it can cause a relapse. In studies, 78% of patients improved when exposed to sunlight, and 77% improved in hot weather. American Indians and native Fijians (many of whom spend a large fraction of their time exposed to sunlight) do not get psoriasis. The disease is uncommon in Afro-Americans and occurs less frequently in the tropics. Studies have shown that elevated body temperature can limit the spread of psoriasis. The highest incidence of psoriasis is found in Caucasians living in colder climates.

The onset of psoriasis can occur as early as a few months after birth... or as late as the seventh decade of life. The average age at onset is twenty-seven.

Women seem to have "flare-ups" during menopause and after pregnancy but the psoriasis lessens or disappears during the pregnancy. When psoriasis begins in the teenage years, its onset usually coincides with puberty.

It is believed that some type of biochemical stimulus triggers the abnormal cell growth that characterizes psoriasis. Psoriasis is considered by some professionals to be an autoimmune disease. According to the *Medical Dictionary for the Non-professional,* autoimmune disease is any of a large group of diseases marked by an abnormality of the functioning of the immune system that causes the production of antibodies against one's own tissues and other body substances.

Most people have skin cells that follow the natural course of growth, taking twenty-eight to thirty days to mature. Psoriasis skin cells, on the other hand, take just three to four days to mature. When we talk about skin cell growth occurring at a much greater-than-normal rate, we are referring to a *metabolic* change. This metabolic change can stop as fast as it starts. In many patients, psoriasis shows up at sites of injuries to the skin.

When a psoriasis lesion clears from the skin it can be hypopigmented (lighter in color than surrounding skin) or hyperpigmented (darker in color than surrounding skin) giving the appearance of a scar. Within time, the normal skin color returns and any evidence of psoriasis will disappear.

During World War II, prisoners confined in German concentration camps found that their attacks of psoriasis ceased. Apparently, starvation slowed the body's metabolism which resulted in the disappearance of the psoriasis.

Psoriasis bleeding occurs because the psoriasis scale is attached to the skin; and when you scrape it off, the fine capillaries that hold and feed it are broken. There is really no other skin problem that looks just like psoriasis.

Sensitive areas of our body, like our face and genital, should be treated with lower strength treatments. These areas are more prone to side-effects. Remember some medications (like steroids) cause a thinning of the skin. Light therapy can be effective but be cautious due to greater risk of burning. But again be cautious since high exposure increases incidence of skin cancer. If you keep sensitive areas and folds of skin dry, it reduces irritation and helps prevent the growth of bacteria and yeast.

In my family, all my siblings, except for my youngest brother, developed psoriasis after the age of thirty. Only two other people in my family in addition to my siblings have psoriasis: my maternal grandmother and my mother. Fortunately, psoriasis has not shown up in any of my siblings' children. My mother has had psoriasis most of her life, although none of her brothers or sisters ever showed any signs of the disease.

My mother is an amazing example of the effect of stress on psoriasis. She had an extremely bad case of psoriasis during most of her adult life. But after she divorced, her psoriasis cleared up and only flares up under great stress and even then, only in a few small patches.

Following is a statement published by Dr. Frederick Lansford, one of a group of doctors and researchers from the Edgar Cayce Foundation, summing up Edgar Cayce's insights into psoriasis:

> *In summary then, it may be said that psoriasis is a disease state in which variable factors reduce the lymph circulation through portions of the gastrointestinal tract causing a thinning of the intestinal walls, usually in the jejunum and/or duodenum, and at times a loss of the villi which aid selective absorption of intestinal contents. As the lesions in the intestines become more pronounced there occurs a seepage or leakage into the circulatory system of toxic substances from the intestinal tract. When the emunctory systems of the body are unable to eliminate these toxic products as fast as they are absorbed, the circulation becomes overburdened and they find their way into the lymph flow of the skin in sufficient quantity to produce congestion and the inflammatory reaction which is characteristic of the disease.*

(From "Commentary on Psoriasis", originally published 11/15/68. Copyright by Edgar Cayce Foundation. Reprinted by permission.)

An article titled "Rx for Psoriasis," appearing in the January 19, 1987 issue of Insight magazine described several aspects of psoriasis:

> *Some doctors believe psoriasis is linked to a disruption in normal cell maturation and growth. Dr. Michael Holick of Tufts University, and his colleague, suspected that the skin of psoriasis patients did not recognize, as well as it should, a hormone produced by the kidney that stops the proliferation of skin cells. (See the chapter on: Vitamins, Minerals and Herbs, for information on the direction in which Dr. Holick took his research.)*

Extreme cases of psoriasis will always require the attention of a medical specialist; however, severe cases are very uncommon.

A general practitioner is a health resource to use when needed. However, according to some in the medical world, 70% to 85%... or as many as 100%... of all known diseases are psychosomatically induced; and, as a result, the majority of medical procedures is unnecessary. This is an important reason to consider alternatives to some standard medical treatments of psoriasis.

Elliott Douglas Derzaph

2 Putting out the Burn: Topical Solutions & Treatments

The skin absorbs and excretes continuously. Whatever you put **in your body** can eventually be eliminated through the pores of your skin. Conversely, the products you put **on your body** can be systematically absorbed. Care should be taken when using prescription topical ointments and creams over long periods of time, because they may be toxic and can be **absorbed into your body**.

Careful removal of psoriatic scales, by hydration (use of water, as in a bath or shower) or by medication to soften the skin, prior to applying other medications, is very important to speed the effect of topical products. The beneficial effects of ointments, creams and oils are reduced if applied to the top layers of existing scales. Treatments should be regularly rotated since it is so easy for our system to become resistant to many types of medications. Gloves, made from plastic often used as disposable kitchen gloves, are handy to use when trying to keep topical solutions on your hands as well as aiding you from scratching yourself at night.

Over the years, I have heard of many unusual topical treatments. One such treatment was used in Kangal, Turkey. It involved allowing live fish to nibble away the psoriasis plaques directly off the human. Apparently it worked to remove the plaques temporarily. However, the feeling of being pinched hard and often was extremely uncomfortable.

I think the most unusual substance I tried on my skin, was suggested by a friend of my brother. The friend had stories of success that convinced me to, once again, try another treatment, even though it sounded somewhat bizarre. If you go to the market you can pick it up tomorrow. That is, if Lamb's fat appeals to you. I find it hard to believe I tried it, but I did. Sometimes the frustration of a disease can make you do silly things. I'm just glad the only side effect was two very greasy bed sheets.

Ointments

Notes in using topical ointments: Don't combine medications; Thick application of medication is not more effective; Chronic use of any steroid product usually diminishes its effectiveness and increases the side-effects; Don't overlap therapies; Irritation may not always mean you're allergic to it; Use the appropriate topical for each location on your body.

In one chapter of his new book, The Best Treatment, Isadore Rosenfeld, M.D. describes a new development in psoriasis treatment and shares his opinions.

> *Psoriasis can be such a miserable business that almost any treatment with some promise should at least be considered. Sulfasalazine (Azulfidine), which is helpful in inflammatory bowel disease and rheumatoid arthritis, also appears to improve psoriasis. It has been reported to result in impressive clearing of the lesions in at least 50% of cases. It's all relatively new, and worth discussing with your dermatologist.*
>
> *There is one additional recent development in the management of psoriasis of which you should be aware. Apparently, in severe cases there is an overproduction of human growth hormone (HGH) by the body. A product called Sandostatin has been shown to decrease the blood levels of HGH, and apparently improve psoriasis. These observations have thus far been made in "uncontrolled" trials, and are currently being tested more scientifically. If your psoriasis is severe, ask your doctor about the status of this Sandostatin research.*

(©1991 The Best Treatment, by Isadore Rosenfeld, M.D. Reprinted by permission.)

(Update: August 1993. Upon contacting a local university and additionally, several local doctors in private practice, I found Sulfasalazine (Azulfidine) had been approved for the treatment of psoriasis - but none of the doctors recommended it. Research on Sandostatin was unknown to these same doctors.)

Oils

I think oils are the most useful and the healthiest items to use on a dry body; you just have to be careful not to get any on your clothes or bedding. Many oils have been used to soothe the itch of psoriasis' dry skin. The most commonly used oils are: almond, coconut, olive, grape seed, castor, aloe, cod liver (fish) oil, lanolin, jojoba, wheat germ and vitamin E. Also, consider pure aloe vera gel, calendula lotion and Egyptian magic cream. The best, in my opinion, is olive oil. Always remember to keep your body away from anything you don't want to get oil on.

Rubbing different types of oil (olive having the best record), on stubborn areas like feet and hands, works for many to clear these areas.

Fish oil, the substance praised by many as reducing heart attack risk, also may find a role in therapy for skin diseases, including psoriasis. Just a few years ago a report from the American Academy of Dermatology indicated that eighteen patients were given fish oil supplements, and improvement in psoriasis was seen in thirteen. *(see Chapter 15: The Natural Approach: Vitamins, Minerals and Herbs, for more information on fish oil.)*

Mud

Mud is another substance I tried, as a result of the recommendation of my younger brother, who obtained good results. He had heard of a spa, in a remote area in the state of Washington, which had been visited by a friend who also had a skin disorder. The spa offered mineral and mud bath self-treatments. My brother obtained the telephone number from his friend and ordered a supply of mud. My brother had a very small area of psoriasis that disappeared after his continuous application of mud for two to three weeks. His psoriasis hadn't returned which was a good year after using the mud.

My mud story is a little different. My brother sent me about a quart of mud from the shipment he received and I followed the directions he gave me. It appeared to have some effect, with a tingling sensation accompanying its use. But after three to four weeks of use without seeing a significant - or even a noticeable - change, I stopped. The daily treatment included the application of the strong smelling mud, followed by a twenty to thirty minute waiting period to allow the mud to dry. The final step was scrubbing it off before going to bed each night and then adding a moisturizer.

Since then I have heard of "Soap Lake" in the state of Washington where many others have visited and had quite a success. The daily regiment uses the stinky mud by applying it liberally on your lesions and leaving it there until it dries, then sunbathing up to an hour followed by a shower and then adding a good moisturizer or oil. A stay of at least two to three weeks appears to provide the best outcome.

Tar

Tar products, which are distilled from coal, are well known to psoriasis patients. Tar can stop the production of skin cells, reduce inflammation, and stop itching and scaling. There are many tar based shampoos available in the marketplace.

Tar is very messy and you have to be careful about going into the sun while tar is on your skin. The most damaging side-effect resulting from prolonged use of tar for some users is skin cancer. You should be sure to take breaks from regular use of tar, and have periodic medical check-ups for skin cancer. Tar remains active on your skin for twenty-four hours after it is applied.

Other Products

In The Doctors Book of Home Remedies published by Rodale Press, Dr. Lawrence Miller says this about psoriasis:

> *"A cold-water bath, maybe with a cup or so of apple cider vinegar added, is great for (the relief of) itching. Another thing that really works is ice, just dump some ice cubes into a small plastic bag and hold it against the afflicted skin. But hot water can make itching worse."*
>
> Dr. Miller also writes about "Zostrix: Hot Stuff for Psoriasis."
>
> Because there is no cure for psoriasis, people scour the planet for treatments and will try anything, including medications designed for other ailments. A good example is Zostrix, an over the counter (O.T.C.) cream used to treat shingles.
>
> *University of Chicago Pritzker, School of Medicine associate professor of clinical pharmacology, Joel Bernstein, M.D., invented (and holds the patent for) Zostrix. It's made from the ingredient in red pepper, capsaicin, that gives real meaning to be word "hot." It's been tested on psoriasis but has been approved by Food and Drug Administration only for shingles, Dr. Bernstein says. "It's unquestionably effective," he claims. "My only concern is that it's a little tricky to use. In fact, if and when it's approved for psoriasis, it will probably be a prescription product."*
>
> *The theory is that Zostrix makes the body exhaust all its supplies of substance P, a chemical that's believed to cause inflammation and is also found in psoriatic plaques. The cream then blocks the body from making more substance F, and it also may prevent proliferation of the blood vessels needed to feed the burgeoning skin cell population in a psoriatic plaque.*
>
> *Zostrix can't be used haphazardly Dr Bernstein cautions. "It won't help unless it's used frequently and continuously for at least three weeks."* And here's the tricky part: *"This stuff burns, and you'd better be prepared for it,"* Dr. Miller says. *It burns your fingers, it burns the plaque, and it will burn your face if you should happen to rub it without first washing off the Zostrix. But the*

burning lessens or vanishes if you keep up the treatments, Dr. Bernstein says.

Our advice: use only with your doctor's approval and close supervision.

(Doctors Book of Home Remedies, ©1990, Rodale Press Inc. Reprinted by permission.)

Dry Skin Brushing

Skin brushing with a natural fiber brush is quite a healthy habit to complement a cleansing program. Skin brushing is a very valuable aid in the release of toxins in the body but only when your psoriasis is not active. **Unfortunately, dry skin brushing is not recommended for most people with psoriasis.** Here are a few comments reprinted from Dr. Linda Berry's book, *Internal Cleansing - A Practical Guide to Colon Health*.

> *Dry skin brushing is one of the best ways to cleanse the skin without removing the protective mantle of acid and oils. Daily skin brushing removes the top layer of dead skin with its build-up of dirt and acid, and deeply cleanses the pores.*
>
> *The skin plays a vital role in ridding the body of toxins and impurities that are potential sources of illness. It has been estimated that the skin eliminates over one pound of waste per day.*
>
> *Skin brushing is one of the most powerful ways to cleanse the lymphatic system. Waste material is carried away from the cells by the blood lymph. Skin brushing stimulates the release of this material from the cells near the surface of the body.*
>
> *Dry skin brushing also stimulates the sweat glands and increases blood circulation to underlying organs and tissues in the body. Today, a sedentary lifestyle and general lack of exercise, along with the common use of antiperspirants, keep people from perspiring enough. As a result, toxins and metabolic waste are not released through sweat as they were intended, but instead, back up into the body. Skin brushing opens up the pores allowing the body to breathe and thus enhances proper functioning of the organs.*
>
> *The best time to skin brush is before your morning shower or bath. Remember to brush when the skin is dry. Brush with one-stroke movements. Use a softer brush for the face. Total brushing should take under three minutes. You will feel an invigorating, tingling sensation over your entire body.*

(From Internal Cleansing - A Practical Guide to Colon Health, by Dr. Linda Berry. Copyright 1985 by Botanica Press. Reprinted by permission.)

Cosmetic Cover-up (cosmeceutical)

Fortunately in today's society there is a wide variety of natural colored, natural ingredient cosmetics which can be used by men and women to conceal normally exposed parts of your skin.

Years ago, I knew a woman who had a bad scar on her face from a car accident. She decided she was comfortable with the scar and didn't bother with make-up. On the other hand, another friend, who had a long scar on her neck from an operation, would at times put makeup on the scar, so it wouldn't be noticed during social events.

Cover-up makeup is different from standard make-up in that it is opaque and waterproof.

In 1992, a new product line named *Dermablend Corrective Cosmetics* was introduced. The Dermablend camouflage system will hide imperfections of all sorts - including psoriasis; yet it looks as natural as your own skin. All Dermablend products are waterproof, long-lasting, non-greasy, smudge-resistant, easy to apply and 100% fragrance-free. Dermablend can be found in most leading department stores. For the store nearest you, write to: Consumer Affairs Director, Dermablend Corrective Cosmetics.

Another company sounding very similar: Covermark Cosmetics, One Anderson Ave., Moonachie, N.J. 07074.

The point to be made in this section is that you should not remove yourself from public activity if the application of cosmetics would create a comfort zone, allowing you to participate.

Other Topical Solutions

The January 1988 issue of Vogue magazine carried an article by Melva Weber titled "Watertight Dressing: Psoriasis Cure." Weber reported on the work of Dr. Stephen J. Friedman, who did a study showing that airtight, watertight adhesive (*hydrocolloid occlusive*) dressings improved, or completely cleared up, psoriasis plaques in a majority of cases.

Hydrocolloid occlusive dressings proved to be as effective as ultraviolet-B treatment. (Ultraviolet-B and other light and radiation treatments are described in a chapter titled: Exposure to Sunshine or Light). Thus, the application of water/moisture is an effective method of clearing up common psoriasis plaques. There was a product available that was using occlusive dressing called "Dermatex Wraps". You apply your medication (non-steroid cream worked best) with disposable plastic bandages with a reusable latex cover and velcro straps. This method normally makes the skin clearer and softer.

Topical solutions are usually more effective and work more quickly if they are confined to the affected area by an occlusive dressing for 12 to 24 hours. Occlusive dressing is made of a polyethylene film similar to the plastic wrap sold in grocery stores, such as Saran Wrap®. Lesions will recur with this therapy. Serious side effects can occur if you are using a toxic, topical solution which is absorbed by the skin. Also, the skin will be unable to breathe and excrete properly over the period of time you wrap your skin. Shorter durations are healthier for your skin but it takes longer for the skin to temporarily relieve itself of psoriasis.

Immediately after getting out of the tub, I use what is known as a shower and bath oil, which is made up of oils and water. Usually I am itch-free for most of the workday. Unless, of course, I let myself get tense, or I consume products that irritate my system during the day.

The most effective use of a topical solution occurs when I can apply the medication while resting, at the end of my day, and then rinse it off before I get into bed. Or when I can apply it prior to bedtime and let it work while I sleep.

During a few tough bouts with psoriasis I used a sauna suit. I wore the suit under my sweats while working out in the gym or running or while working around the house. Sometimes I would sleep with the suit on, but around 3:00 a.m. my discomfort threshold would usually be exceeded and I would have to arise to take the suit off. I noticed favorable results, although you should watch that you don't overdue the use of the suit. Also, my suit kept tearing. The sauna suit had the side benefit of removing a few pounds from my body.

Psoria-Gard® skin treatment system is purported to be the latest breakthrough formula. Developed over a 15 year period, Hobe Laboratories, Inc., of Phoenix created a natural ingredient based treatment. The manufacturer claims this topically applied material will quickly relieve and control the redness, itching and scaling associated with psoriasis.

Exorex has a Holistic based treatment Psoriasis Clinic located near Cape Town, South Africa. The clinic offers total privacy and tranquility, peace and quiet, sights and sounds of abundant wildlife, a fun, stress-free, and access to a variety of recreational facilities, a twelve day program with psoriasis trained medical personnel treating the physical and psychological effects. They offer expert evaluation, education and care and a support program for when you return home.

Skin-Cap

Skin-Cap - A product that worked effectively for many has been pulled off the market since 1997 in the U.S. and Canada. The steroid (clobetasol) that was not listed by the manufacturer or distributors anywhere turns out to be a prescription product with powerful side effects.

Skin-Cap (April 1999 report) product contains clobetasol propionate, a prescription steroid medication. A very effective product in clearing psoriasis but some suffer severe adverse skin reactions from its use if not used appropriately. (NPF reported over 100 cases of severe adverse reactions). Most people stated it cleared psoriasis better than any other product out.

I had never wanted to endorse any product in my life. However, Skin-Cap, an OTC (over-the-counter [non-prescription]) product, almost became an exception. I came upon this product in a small ad in a local newspaper. I sent for information and was impressed by the claims and testimonials. I immediately ordered two aerosol canisters and their shampoo.

I jumped right in giving it a test run, using the spray once each morning before getting dressed, and once each evening between the completion of my work and bedtime. I had my wife participate, for convenience, encouragement and her observations (we all know the frustrations!). Within a week, we noticed a change and before a month had passed most of the psoriasis on my body had disappeared.

Of all the products I've used, I believed this was the best by far. Statistics show success with over 75% of patients reporting either "good" or "very good" results. Less than 4% have indicated failure to obtain relief. A month's treatment for many is a minimum of $50. This is truly a non-messy and convenient product to use and transport. Plus, the supplier did offer a 100% money back guarantee. Who thought we would ever find such a product? Until an actual cure gets here (probably when we have breakthrough in both genetics and Emotional Intelligence®), I thought I couldn't be recommending a better product to satisfy the needs of psoriasis sufferers. Then the news came out from the FDA... the product has a steroid.

But here are the details in case someone finds a solution that allows a way for us to use it. Skin-Cap is used for any itchy flaking red skin. It is available as colorless, odorless, stain free, aerosol, and also as a shampoo. It relieves the flaking, itching and redness characteristic of psoriasis.

Skin-Cap's active ingredient is zinc pyrithione and a steroid, which, according to the supplier, exerts an antibacterial and antifungal action, mainly on the Pityrosporum ovale and Pityrosporum orgiculare, achieving a potent inhibition of certain saprophyte flora in the cornea layer through an antiproliferative cytostatic effect.

I sure hope that a very thorough analysis is done of Skin-Cap and a newer version is re-presented to the public. I have never been more satisfied with the results of any product like I was with Skin-Cap. We had found an effective product for psoriasis. Now we need to find a way to make it safe to use.

Many new sprays have entered the market since Skin-Cap arrived with many of them using the zinc pyrithione as the main active ingredient. Cleariasis skin therapy spray, by Skin-Tech, goes another direction and uses purified liquid coal tar.

Ontos Inc. created Noble Formula in spray or cream a zinc pyrithione and sodium laurly sulfate and states a 60% improvement. Also, they have Noble Formula Rx which has a steroid (Clobetasol) and states a 90% improvement. The Rx product must be ordered with a prescription through Ontos. This product appears to be the closest alternative to Skin-Cap that I am aware of at this time, but, more research is needed.

So keep in mind some topical basics: Do not combine medications without professional guidance; a thin application of medication is all that is needed; try the "pulse therapy" which is when you use strong topical corticosteroids on weekends and nonsteroidal antipsoratic agents during the weekdays which lessens side effects and extends the medications use before its effect diminishes (lack of response); limit use of steroids to face, groin and armpits; use different medications for different areas which ever is the best choice for each area.

3 Letting the Sun Shine In: Exposure to Sunshine or Light

I had just returned from my honeymoon and recalled an interesting occurrence. During the two weeks I spent on the island of Kauai, I was in the saltwater and sun every day; and my psoriasis stopped itching and flaring up. But when I got to Oahu and ceased both my daily swim in the ocean and my relaxation in the sun, my psoriasis began to itch and flare up again.

The sun heats our skin, increasing blood flow and circulation, which helps our body fight infection, in turn, increasing our white blood cell count. Natural sunlight has a clearing effect in 80% of patients with moderate exposure. As with most aids to psoriasis, you must be **patient, consistent and persistent**. A gradual tan is suggested, acquired from periods of short duration exposure to the sun. If you burn, instead of tanning, your psoriasis will worsen temporarily (the degree depends on the individual).

The application of sun screen is recommended to control burning and allow tanning, especially between 11:00 a.m. and 3:00 p.m. when the sun is very nearly overhead and therefore at its strongest. If you are not using a sun screen at least use a moisturizer. Many people state that exposure to sunshine on a regular basis keeps their psoriasis away. Be sure to use sunglasses to protect your eyes from (UVA and UVB) *ultraviolet radiation*.

Please check with your healthcare provider/doctor before beginning to expose yourself to any light treatment even tanning in the sun especially in the length of time you can be in the sun in your part of the world. Use caution to ensure you don't overdue the time in the sun. Recommendations by experts is to sunbathe at least three times a week for short periods using a thin layer of some type of moisturizing product.

The *Dead Sea treatment* (a form of climatotherapy) has long been used by patients from around the world. The treatment combines sunshine and saltwater for up to six hours a day over a period of three to four weeks. Note, however, that saltwater can sting or be quite irritating to active psoriasis.

Studies show that the large majority of psoriasis sufferers coming to the Dead Sea for treatment show significant improvement. One recent study showed 56% cleared and another 29% showed excellent improvement. The time span before the reappearance of psoriasis ranges from one to twelve months. Many psoriasis sufferers visit the Dead Sea twice a year, for two week periods, and claim to stay clear. The sea has a high mineral content, a very high salt content, a higher oxygen and bromine concentration than most bodies of water, and no living microorganisms. The sunlight in that geographical area also has high levels of UVA. And, you are in a very stress free and relaxing environment.

UVA is longwave ultraviolet radiation that causes the melanin in the **surface of the skin** to oxidize and turn brown. UVA is the part of "sunlight" which causes tanning. UVA radiation and the drug, *psoralen*, when combined in therapy, is known as PUVA. The treatment can clear a patient for periods ranging from a few weeks to more than a year. Treatment is effective in at least 80% of cases and some patients can stay clear for up to three years. The average length of treatment is thirty sessions, but many more may be needed. People who are sun-sensitive can use this treatment.

PUVA can cause many side-effects including minor itching, nausea, worsening of psoriasis, depression, skin cancer and cataracts. PUVA in some people causes thickening and darkening of hair and can cause a deep, burning itch that can last weeks to months. Only individuals suffering from severe psoriasis, with coverage of 30% or more, should consider PUVA as a treatment.

Research has shown that genital tumors have occurred 50 times the expected incidence when compared to the general population with people who received PUVA treatment. Therefore for early detection be sure to get genital screening soon after any treatment and continue regular ongoing screening.

UVB is shortwave ultraviolet radiation that stimulates melanin production **within the skin**. The melanin travels to the surface of the skin in a form known as granules. UVB is the part of "sunlight" that exposure to Sunshine or Light causes sunburns. UVB therapy is called phototherapy and can temporarily clear psoriasis. Clearance can last from a week to more than a year. On the average twenty to thirty sessions are needed to clear psoriasis. Tar is applied prior to the exposure to UVB. The use of baths and moisturizers, such as oils or vaseline, instead of tar, have also proven to be helpful.

Side effects range from temporary worsening of the psoriasis to skin cancer. In severe cases of psoriasis the Goeckerman regiment is used. This treatment involves very concentrated uses of tar and UVB over a three to four week period.

The following is abstracted from The New England Journal of Medicine.

Phototherapy and Photochemotherapy

It should be noted that PUVA and ultraviolet B radiation cause damage to membranes as well as to DNA, and this will induce cell death. In addition, ultraviolet A rays penetrate much farther into the dermis than ultraviolet B rays. Thus, PUVA's potential effect on the dermal vasculature and cellular infiltrates is greater than that of ultraviolet B radiation. PUVA can also alter immune responses.

(From The New England Journal of Medicine (NEJM), by John H. Epstein, M.D., Vol. 322, No. 16, p. 1150, April 19, 1990, copyright 1990. Reprinted by permission.)

For persistent cases of psoriasis many doctors recommend the patient buy a portable ultraviolet lamp ("sunlamp") and give him/herself treatments at home on a regular basis. Timed exposures usually begins at about 2 minutes and increase a few seconds daily. Taking a tar bath prior to use increases the effectiveness of the treatment.

Narrow-band UVB therapy. Parts of the world have used this new treatment for years. Studies have shown faster clearing and more complete disease resolution with this new therapy that falls between broad-band and PUVA. It works better, more quickly and patients are finding it easy to do than standard UVB therapy and believed to be less risky than PUVA, no psoralen pills or wearing protective sunglasses up to 24 hours after treatment either. Patients get three narrow-band UVB treatments a week, and they can expect clearing in six-to-eight weeks. Treatments can usually stop after a two-week maintenance dose. Narrow-band UVB do not expose the skin to wavelengths of light that are known to be cancer-causing.

Finding a treatment center with the new equipment can be a challenge due to the new costs, the relative effectiveness and the new status of the therapy. Also, a little extra care is necessary because burning is more common.

Care when using UV light equipment is essential, especially with regard to choosing the proper eye-wear to protect the eyes. The sunlamp should have an **automatic timer**. Fluorescent type lamps are better overall but are bulky.

More information can be obtained from "Safer and More Successful Suntanning," by the editors of *Consumer Guide*, available in most libraries. Be sure to check with your doctor before using a sunlamp while taking any drug (especially lithium or beta-blockers) because of the possibility of interactions.

During the winter, when I couldn't find any sunlight, I found that visiting a local tanning salon once a week, aided in keeping my psoriasis in check. Since then I have purchased a home unit. Sessions of 10 to 20 minutes in length were good for my skin type. Though each person must work with their care-giver to find the optimum time for each piece of equipment available.

For those individuals that have the money and space they can bring a full length fluorescent lamp bed into their home (or they may have an insurance company that pays for the equipment). If you are so lucky, be sure to buy fluorescent tubes that produce the appropriate wavelengths for psoriasis patients. When choosing equipment for home use, or when at tanning salons, be sure to select units built especially for psoriasis or select lamps producing high UVA and low UVB.

Guidelines exist for usage of home phototherapy systems. Some manufacturers require a doctor's prescription for purchase. Insurance policies vary with regard to coverage of equipment cost for home use.

Be sure to check with your doctor when considering the use of home or salon type units. Without proper medical advice, you could receive less than a therapeutic dose, or alternatively, burn yourself causing pain and extreme irritation.

PSORALENS

Psoralens/photosensitizers increase the reactivity of the skin to ultraviolet and/or visible radiation. When ultraviolet radiation strikes the photosensitzer in the skin, a complex phototoxic reaction occurs. The reaction occurs in a sunburn.

PUVA which is Psoralens and UVA therapy is usually highly effective in treating extensive psoriasis. Psoralens also effect the human eye and can cause eye damage and cataract formation. Be sure to wear protective eyeware for at least 24 hours after PUVA treatment. Pregnant women are recommended not to have PUVA.

Coal tar is well-known as a photosensitizer and contains more than 25 different chemicals that are individual photosensitizers. A well-known and possibly the ultimate photosensitizer is psoralen, along with its derivatives. Psoralens are activated in the skin by UVA which normally tans people.

Psoralens are available in a wide variety of foods - figs, parsley, celery, parsnips, angelica, bergamont, rue, dill, fennel, carrots, lemon, queen anne lace, giant hogweed, lime and cloves.

4 Refreshed by Water: The Benefits of H2O

The most healthy product a human can consume is water. Pure, clean, refreshing drinking water is a truly satisfying fluid the body needs. Just as the insides of our bodies need water to thrive, the outsides of our bodies stay healthier when clean water is applied regularly.

We have a tendency, after we wash our bodies, to rub them dry with a towel. Rubbing is harsh and removes too much of the water that is so healthy for the body. So, use the towel to pat your skin dry instead.

Water evaporates faster from the skin of people with psoriasis than from the skin of those who don't have the disease. When moisturizers and oils are put on the body after bathing, they work as a baffle to prevent the moisture/water from escaping and thus bring relief from dry skin and scaling. Also, remember that moisturizers have few, if any, side-effects as compared to most topical medications. Reapplying a moisturizer throughout the day is of great benefit and relief.

Most of the body's water loss occurs in one of two ways: *excretion*, in the form of urine, which accounts for 50% of water loss, and *secretion*, in the form of perspiration, which accounts for 31% of water loss. Maintaining skin that is clean and has adequate moisture is paramount when psoriasis is part of your life. People who live in colder and/or drier climates, may want to install humidifiers or vaporizers in their homes, to reduce skin discomfort.

Water in many forms is enjoyable and soothing to psoriasis patients. Try a few of the following:

- Swimming in fresh water

- Soaking in a Jacuzzi

- Swimming in saltwater

- Sitting in a steam room

- Soaking in a tub

- Immersing in a mud bath

Be cautious when trying the above - make sure that the water/steam is not too hot and that the chlorine level is not so great as to cause drying.

Many soaps have a drying effect on the skin. Be sure to wash off all soap after a shower or a bath.

I sometimes use sea-salt in a warm tub as an alternative to soaking in the ocean. It is best not to leave saltwater on the skin. Showering is suggested after your dip in the ocean or a bath with sea-salt. Always use a moisturizer after a soak.

Swimming in a pool or sitting in a Jacuzzi is great for your skin as long as you remove any chlorine by taking a shower when you are finished. Follow a shower with the application of a moisturizer. The quicker you apply the moisturizer the more moisture you trap and the healthier your skin. Waiting just a few minutes can cause much of the moisture to evaporate thus rendering the moisturizer useless; so make the application of a moisturizer your first task after you get out of the tub or shower.

Since so many places put chlorine or other harsh chemicals into the water it is to your benefit to buy and use water filters. Filters come as simple as singular drinking or shower water filters to whole house filtering systems.

Dry skin brushing *(see Chapter 2: Putting Out the Burn: Topical Solutions & Treatments)* before a shower allows a deeper and more thorough cleansing of the skin. Do not brush if the skin is, or becomes, irritated. Do not brush psoriatic plaques.

Occlusive dressing *(see Chapter 2: Putting Out the Burn: Topical Solutions & Treatments)* with applied topicals from water to steroids can soften the plaques for easy non-damaging removal.

5 Savoring your Life: Massage

Massage allows a psoriasis sufferer to be touched (a need that can increase, during outbreaks). Use of oils can reduce skin irritation and be quite soothing to your dry skin. Your muscles can be relaxed allowing relief from tensions, a primary and essential benefit to psoriasis sufferers.

The skin contains more than five million receptors that transmit messages to the brain. Massage promotes the flow of lymphatic fluid, lowers levels of stress hormones, and boosts productive endorphins, the body's natural painkillers.

The Chinese have used massages to treat bodily imbalances by enhancing the flow of "chi," the body's vital energy.

Massages vary almost as much as personality types. **French massage** is light and uses a powder. **Swedish massage** is deep and uses oils. Lymphatic is a term that denotes a medium massage which stimulates the secretion of toxic wastes. **Polarity massage** is light, is often a complement to other massages and is designed to put the body's energy field into balance.

Lymphatic and polarity massages are gentle and relaxing and help to reduce stress.

The lymphatic system runs throughout the body and its proper functioning is vital to a healthy system. The lymphatic system consists of channels with one-way valves transporting lymph fluid in clusters. The lymph nodes along these channels act as traps to arrest the spread of infections. Lymphatic massages stimulate the secretion of toxic wastes, eliminating stagnant body fluids. The body tissue is cleansed and nourished at a cellular level.

I have enjoyed many pleasurable hours on the tables of good massage practitioners. I would venture to say that many of us have been ecstatic after receiving a back or neck or foot massage for even just a few minutes. Most of us have experienced the pleasure of receiving a massage, but we seldom participate in providing its pleasure. All forms of massage are quite enjoyable and rewarding, though I prefer the deeper muscle massage, using plenty of coconut oil.

On several occasions I have had the pleasure of experiencing the professional skills of Joan, a massage practitioner in Southern California. Joan gave me a typewritten sheet containing the following general overview on lymphatic massage.

Elliott Douglas Derzaph

Massage - A Natural High!

Regular massage can have a profound effect on the physical and emotional well-being. It also has a positive effect on appearance. After only a few weeks of regular massage, the remarkable results of this ancient art will be noticed.

Massage stimulates nerve supply and cell activity. Blood and lymph is passed more efficiently through the body, allowing a replenishment of these vital fluids. The work of the heart is lessened due to improvement in surface circulation and there is an increase in the number of red and white blood cells. Lactic acid is removed from stiff overworked muscles, preventing cramping and muscle spasm and in addition, endorphins, a natural chemical which creates relaxation and relief of pain and a general sense of well-being, are produced.

Physiologically - Massage can **lessen or eliminate**:

- Back, neck and shoulder pain
- Migraine, tension and sinus headaches
- Eyestrain
- Hypertension (high blood pressure)
- Arthritis and bursitis pain
- Sore and stiff muscles
- Muscle spasms and cramps
- Muscle atrophy
- Indigestion and menstrual discomfort

Cosmetically - Massage can **lessen or eliminate**:

- Wrinkles
- Cellulite

Cosmetically - Massage can **improve**:

- Posture
- Body awareness
- Body image
- Muscle tone
- Fat loss, by 10-15%, for dieters
- Skin tone and texture

Psychologically - Massage can **lessen or eliminate**:

- Anxiety
- Depression
- Emotional blocks
- Touch deprivation
- Feelings of isolation and loneliness
- Tiredness and lack of energy
- Drug and alcohol abuse

Psychologically - Massage can **increase**:

- Sensuality
- Contentment
- Pleasure and happiness
- A feeling of well-being

The Massage Practitioner who is centered, empathetic and intuitive also benefits considerably from this practice, as it not only creates a meditative peace, but the contact and exercise bring about physiological and psychological restoration.

I think everyone agrees that a good massage is a valuable contribution to overall good health and in improving how we feel. As I was typing this into my computer I got a strong urge to pick up the phone and make an appointment. I cannot think of a better way to treat myself after a hard work week.

Elliott Douglas Derzaph

6 The Last Resort: Surgery

I have read, and heard firsthand, many stories about unnecessary surgical procedures. Two recent articles are described below to give you an idea of the importance of self-knowledge to your health.

1) An article appearing in the March 22, 1990 issue of *The Wall Street Journal*, titled "A.M.A., Rand Go After Modern Ill: Unneeded Procedures," by Ron Winslow and Sonia L. Nazario.

    Unnecessary procedures compromise the quality of care and add billions to the U.S. health costs. Rand estimated more than $50 billion a year is added to the nation's health bill for unneeded procedures.

2) An article appearing in the April 16, 1989 issue of *The New York Times* (magazine), titled "Unnecessary Surgery," by James Barron.

    Congress House Investigation Committee found that even as far back as 1975 two million unjustified operations were performed in Medicaid and Medicare programs at a cost of $4 billion.

This information is presented to demonstrate that caution, knowledge and at least two, preferably three, medical opinions should be considered before proceeding with surgery. Medical care that is non-invasive is recommended when choices are available. Always discuss all available options with your doctor before making a decision.

The following is a commentary on a non-invasive procedure taken from an article in a 1987 issue of *Insight* magazine.

> *Dr. Robert Skinner, a dermatologist at the University of Tennessee at Memphis, is treating psoriasis patients by using a laser beam to burn away the scaly patch as well as an ultrathin layer of skin beneath it. The precision of the laser allows removal of the patches without scarring or damaging the healthy tissue. Over the past eight months, eight patients have had the laser treatment; so far, only one has had a recurrence of the condition.*
>
> *Skinner and his colleagues suggest that the laser beams destroy not only the scaly patches of skin but also bacteria or yeast*

microorganisms trapped in the skin that trigger an immune response, which causes the skin to develop the itchy scales. Seven years ago, University of Tennessee researchers proposed this theory on the cause of psoriasis, and doctors say the success of laser treatment lends support to the theory, since the laser would burn away the bacteria as well as the skin.

(From an article in *Insight* magazine, by Katie Tyndall, issue of March 30, 1987. Copyright 1987. Reprinted by permission.)

In a letter from Dr. Skinner dated 7/20/93: The lesions did not recur after the surgery sites healed. Some of these patients were examined in a 6-8 year follow-up, and the lesions still had not recurred even though they had developed psoriasis in other areas of the body. This treatment has not gained wide acceptance, because it is primarily for someone with a few stable lesions, and it is not a good treatment for someone with widespread psoriasis or continually active psoriasis.

Lasers use high intensity narrow band radiation to destroy cells of the scales or the attached blood vessels. Types available are - Alexandrite, Carbon dioxide, C-beam (pulsed dye) and Excimer. Lasers appear to have one of the longest remission periods of up to 13 months.

Photo dynamic therapy is another use of laser light; it involves the use of a photosensitive drug derived from animals. PUVA, described in the chapter on: Exposure to Sunshine or Light involves the plant derived drug psoralen. *(see Chapter 3: Letting the Sun shine in: Exposure to Sunshine or Light.)*

Extract from Fall 1998 Canadian Psoriasis Foundation NL Volume 13 No. 3 an article titled "Are lasers a treatment option of psoriasis?" Last year a study was completed at the University of British Columbia Division of Dermatology in which patients with psoriasis participated, with three different lasers. In this study comparisons were made of the pulsed-dye laser (up to three separate treatments), the carbon dioxide laser (one treatment only), and the alexandrite laser (up to three separate treatments).

The carbon dioxide laser used in our study was an improved version that utilized a computer-driven scanning system to minimize the risk of scarring. The study was restricted to patients with long-standing psoriasis and in each patient only one or two plaques were selected for laser surgery. All patients underwent treatment on an outpatient basis at the Lions Laser Skin Centre of the Vancouver General Hospital.

The results showed that compared to no-laser controls, (in which a portion of a plaque is left untreated for comparison purposes), the carbon dioxide and pulsed-dye lasers were consistently effective for psoriasis, whereas the alexandrite laser was not reliably effective.

Improvement could be seen as early as two months after the start of treatment and persisted for this six-month duration of the official follow-up period. A few of the treated sites have remained clear of psoriasis for over one year following laser surgery.

One treatment with the carbon dioxide laser was as good as two or three treatments with the pulsed-dye laser. What was also interesting was the fact that lasers targeting different components of the skin led to the same degree of improvement in psoriasis. In other words, whether it was the carbon dioxide laser selectively vaporizing the top layers of the skin or the pulsed-dye laser altering the abnormal psoriatic blood vessels, the results were the same.

The laser surgery was well tolerated by the participants in the study. The treatment of psoriasis with lasers is still considered experimental by many, but this study has demonstrated that additional research on lasers for psoriasis is warranted.

In November 2001, news came out through the NPF about the Xtrac excimer laser from PhotoMedex. They have a laser which concentrates only on active lesions for mild to moderate cases of psoriasis. There is no risk of healthy skin being damaged and it takes a few minutes in as little as four sessions to get results that typically last a few months.

In National Psoriasis Foundation N.L. Jan/Feb 2002 it reported that Pulsed dye lasers were getting approximately 60% improvements with psoriasis plaques. Also, a new device called "C-beam Laser" is available just for people with psoriasis.

Laser treatment is painful unless an anesthetic is used. It has been known to cause bruising, blistering, scarring or pigment changes.

Cryotherapy

In limited usage when other treatments don't work some doctors will try cryotherapy using liquid nitrogen (a very cold substance) to assist in the removal of small psoriasis plaques. Liquid nitrogen freezes the skin producing a blister that takes several weeks to heal and the skin to become clear.

7 Caring for Hair, Nails and Ears

I find that a few minutes of gentle scalp massage (not scraping) aids healing in psoriasis. When my scalp is very dry or has thick scales I apply an oil during the massage. Just enough oil is used to moisten and remove the itch. When a modest amount of oil is used, you'll find it easy to wash out when you shower. If you are applying it at bedtime, lay an old towel across your pillow to absorb the excess oil so it does not damage your bedding.

Many psoriasis patients think scalp psoriasis will cause loss of hair - but it doesn't. Psoriasis affects the external skin and not the internal layers where hair roots originate. Most of the hair products that help control scalp psoriasis are tar based shampoos. Drugstores and supermarkets usually carry several brands of tar shampoos. Pharmacists are helpful in recommending the most effective brands, to ease persistent itching, and for treating scalp psoriasis.

Shaving when your skin is irritated can exacerbate your psoriasis so when you must shave areas of where psoriasis is active shave down, only one stroke and only one direction.

Gelatin, biotin, sulfur, iodine, cysteine, vitamin C, vitamin A, vitamin B complex and a multivitamin-mineral complex are all recommended for healthy hair and nails. You can buy gelatin in capsules or in powdered form, natural or orange flavored, in supermarkets and health food stores. If you wish to harden your nails and keep them from breaking easily, you can use any of several products including PsoriNail™ and Onyplex™ or a non-gloss clear nail polish, though none is likely to produce normal looking nails. Another product recently suggested is Special Nail Preparation, made with acetyl mandelic acid; I have not tried this product myself.

Psoriasis of the nails is the least noticeable in its progression, as compared with all other forms of psoriasis. Through the "grapevine," I heard that stimulating the area above the nails would prevent nail damage from becoming extensive. Since then, I have used a small, natural fiber brush on the nail area of my hands whenever I bathe. My nails have never returned to their original clear, smooth shape; but I have noticed that my nails look much less pitted and damaged than they were before I started this practice. For some, nail cleaning can cause trauma or promote separation of the nail bed and should be avoided.

Nails are difficult to treat. Finger nails take a year and toe nails two years to completely grow out. Keep the nails trimmed back to where the nails are firmly attached; Wear gloves when working; Soak the nails in oils or moisturizers (the softening makes trimming easier); Apply nail hardener or polish. Nails afflicted with psoriasis may get some help from rubbing Vick's Vapo-Rub® ointment twice a day. Some people have had success with a similar product on their overall skin by using Campho-phenique.

Do you have a nail fungus? Nail fungus can be the cause of your nail damage. "Nail Restoration Clinic" is the name of a U.S. company located in Southern California which offers a new method of external treatment which it claims "no pain, no pills and no surgery." The cost just for your first office visit can be $100 before beginning any therapy.

EARS

Ears need to be worked with very carefully. I got ear infections every couple of years and my doctor recommended using a large 30cc syringe with a plastic tip to inject warm water slowly and carefully into the ear facing towards the sink. The idea is to wash out the ear completely of any particles. Do not stick the tip into your ear canal. Repeat the flushing of each ear with 4 to 7 syringes full of water. I find that this is an effective tool to get rid of any psoriasis residues in the ear canal.

Be sure to **hold the syringe firmly** in one hand while injecting the water into your ear. Please be careful.

8 How to Dress functionally with Psoriasis

Clothing is important to the human body. Besides keeping us warm and protecting us against the elements, clothing is a tool of many uses - from mating to the display of power. Some even become slaves to their compulsions to continually buy new clothes.

Clothing is one area most of us don't consider when making choices that might benefit our health. Natural fibers feel more comfortable because natural material breathes more than synthetics. Also, it is quite important to avoid the residues of certain chemicals that are used in manufacturing or cleaning clothing. The skin of some people can become quite irritated when chemicals in clothing touch their bodies. I had to give up starching my shirts because the starch irritated my skin. I found a good pressing to be sufficient for all my dress shirts.

People with psoriasis have specific needs that may be different from those of non-sufferers. Over 40 percent in a recent survey said that their psoriasis affect their clothing choices. They need clothes that are comfortable, clothes that don't itch, clothes that effectively keep the harsh elements away from their sensitive skin. There is nothing more annoying than causing additional discomfort to skin that is "naturally" itchy, by wearing clothing that irritates the skin.

Special methods are needed to clean clothes laden with the residue of topical treatment products. Add an 8 ounce box of baking soda to the wash to help remove oils from the clothing.

Fabrics include those made of natural fibers as well as those made of one or more of a multitude of synthetics. I find natural fibers to be the best choice by far. Synthetics seem to cause more itching than clothes made of cotton, linen or silk. I find that even wool can be worn if a lining is used by those who find direct contact gives them discomfort.

In some places in Canada and Great Britain some men use "pant liners" to prevent the itching that can result from contact with wool. Pant liners could be likened to a paper thin pair of pants or thermal underwear ("long johns"); to some they might look more like boxer shorts with pant legs. In warmer weather, a thin material is normally used, whereas, during the colder, winter months you can use regular thermal underwear. I gave up wearing wool for many years until I happened upon the pant liners. Pant liners are made from a variety of fabrics but most are made of cotton. I also discovered a secondary use for the pant liners; shielding my good clothes from the ointments and oils used on my skin.

Dress shirts have been part of my daily attire for years. Unfortunately, I had to throw away quite a few shirts before they wore out because they were stained by the oils and other substances I put on my skin. I soon realized it was cheaper to use an undershirt, instead of a good white shirt, to absorb excess oil or ointment.

There is a new fabric (four way stretch lycra™) that is opaque to the eye, but which allows ultraviolet light to pass through and tan the skin underneath. The penetration is equivalent to that resulting after the application of tanning lotion with an SPF of 10. This would allow a person with psoriasis to tan with little or no embarrassment. Initially only swimsuits were made of this material but other articles of clothing are being made as interest grows. The swimsuits are also known as "non-tan line swimsuits." The manufacturers of these type of swimsuits are Coolware Co. Inc. and Lifestyles Direct.

Also, Coolware manufactures a product similar called Cooltan® shirts. These tan-through shirts, made of 100% cotton, can be machine washed and air dried. This light weight fabric (micro sol) has an SPF-6 sunscreen equivalent and will keep you cooler and drier. This company has expressed interest, if there is enough demand, in producing a complete clothing line for people shy about public exposure.

In the meantime, mesh or netting-type tops can allow a fair amount of sun on the skin while not allowing excessive visual exposure. Some sporting goods stores carry shirts designed to be worn under wet-suits; but these shirts could also be worn by themselves when swimming in public. These shirts are also designed to keep the user warm, thus fulfilling two needs.

Gloves made of plastic or latex can be useful to wear to cover medication which you have applied. Further, you do not want it to rub off on anything or create the occlusive dressing affect. To hide a bad case of psoriasis of the hands you may want to wear sports gloves usually made of leather with the fingers cut out just above the second knuckle. A benefit of wearing these type of gloves is it gives people the impression you are into sports.

Cleaning blood stains from clothes can easily be remedied by brushing hydrogen peroxide on it. Use caution to check a small area of the material as to staining first.

9 Physical Activity benefits your overall Health as well as helping to control Psoriatic Arthritis

The key to good health will always include a balanced diet, physical activity and an emotional and intellectual participation and appreciation for what life offers.

In order to maintain good physical health you must be active. If the activity is enjoyable it will not only help you maintain a healthy body, but it will be emotionally satisfying and the likelihood that you will drop the activity because of boredom is reduced. We all know that if your emotions support you, you will make the necessary effort. Always keep a keen eye open for reasons to be active.

While being active, keep whatever muscles are not being used, relaxed. You should also relax your mind. It is refreshing to the mind and body to have a break from their normal activities. If you allow yourself to absorb whatever nature offers you... a breeze, the sky, trees, grass, rain or any other face of nature - the appreciation will increase the pleasure of your outdoor activities.

The minimum amount of physical exertion/activity you should engage in is a period of thirty minutes, three times a week, every week or fifteen minutes a day. Just to get you going start with just five minutes every day. Everyone should consider diversity in their activities. A few recommended activities:

- Deep Breathing
- Isometrics
- Walking
- Swimming
- Rowing
- Running
- Stretching
- Yoga
- Dancing
- Tai Chi
- Martial Arts
- Rope Skipping
- Trampoline
- Bicycling
- Skiing
- Gymnastics

The machines with the most consistent usage is the motorized treadmill followed by strength-training machines. Do whichever activities you enjoy to stay active.

A beneficial side effect of regular and challenging exercise programs is the production of endorphins. Studies have shown that many people who are unhealthy have low endorphin levels. At Case Western Reserve University, Dr. Charles Denko measured endorphin levels in the blood of patients. Endorphin levels were low in patients with diseases including arthritis, gout, and psoriasis. Dr. Denko suggested that the endorphins are part of man's protective mechanisms for fighting inflammation. If this is the case, a low level of endorphins may make it harder for a person to resist inflammation. All people who suffer from psoriasis should make the effort to be active regularly, and receive the health benefits.

Any type of aerobic exercise improves the body's health by supplying blood carrying oxygen to the muscles which increase the cell's capacity to use oxygen, being the most important product in a healthy body.

The key to keeping fit is having a positive attitude towards exercise. You should develop a fitness exercise program that is easy to maintain as well as enjoyable, whether it's dancing or brisk walking. You should tailor a program to match your personality and which is ***easily incorporated into your daily schedule.*** I think the terms "aerobic & flexibility sparks" clarify the most up-to-date view of keeping healthy by daily incorporating some physical vigor.

Exercising on your own, rather than going to an outside facility, such as a gym, is highly recommended. This will ensure that you achieve your goal without distractions. Keep in mind that the main objective in exercising is to remain or become healthy by strengthening your muscles, including your heart, and improving your level of endurance.

Yoga tones the muscles, balances all parts of the body, increases flexibility, creates deep relaxation, is a stress reducer, increases cardiovascular efficiency, creates bone and muscle strength, gives range of motion, reduces risk of injury in other activities, as well as it improves respiration, posture, balance, coordination and concentration. Yoga can be started by taking a few classes to learn the basics correctly. Varied health facilities offer classes. Wear comfortable clothes, bring a mat and try to attend once a week.

When exercising it is important that you check your pulse. Your pulse rate reflects your physical and even your emotional condition; it is the best measure of the body's overall condition.

Check what your pulse rate should be, resting and active, with your doctor, or a health facilities director. Many health clubs display this information on wall charts using your age and weight as overall guides.

Your pulse may easily be taken at the wrist or neck. Most people prefer taking their pulse by using the pad of the middle finger. Press lightly against the radial artery in your wrist, just inside your wrist bone at the base of your thumb joint or on the left or right side of the Adam's apple. Take the pulse *immediately* after your activity to get a true reading of your exertion; your pulse drops very rapidly after activity ceases. The easiest method of getting an accurate reading is to count for fifteen seconds and multiply by four.

If you decide to use yoga as your path to a healthy body - and in particular a healthy spine - try the five simple exercises offered in the book, *Ancient Secret of the Fountain of Youth* by Peter Kelder. The complete exercise program takes just five to ten minutes to complete. The exercises include different forms of stretching and cover all the major muscle groups of the body. This type of workout will keep all the muscles active and stretched while maintaining a fluid spine. The author recommends pacing the number of repetitions in a workout period to match your lifestyle and current physical condition.

Arthritis

The common symptoms of arthritis include stiffness, pain and swelling in and around the joints, also it may manifest in morning sickness and tiredness, or reduced range of motion in joint. Psoriatic arthritis primarily targets the soft tissues around the joints, such as the ligaments, tendons and bursae (fluid-lined sacs that prevent friction). Psoriatic arthritis can target the joint closest to the tips of the fingers and toes, called the distal joints.

Often arthritis begins between the ages of 30 and 50.

Being physically active and an eating program geared toward arthritic relief is the easiest and apparently the most effective program.

Some people have gotten relief from either eating a particular food or not eating a particular food. The following are ones that some have benefitted from:

- Certo (1 tbsp) and unsweetened grape juice (8 ounces) a day
- Gelatin - two envelopes Knox Gelatin daily in hot water
- Dwou Hwau Tea - tea
- White Flower Balm - topical
- Collastin - natural nutritional solution for pain (capsule)
- Zostrix - (hot) topical cream with capsaicin

- Glucosamine+MSM - capsule
- CartazyneDS system - natural pill
- Gluco-Gel - naturopathy capsule
- Glucosamine and Chondrotin sulfates - nutritional pills

ARTHRITIS DRUGS (examples):

    Arave (leflunomide) - second-line therapies
    Enbrel (etanercept) - second-line therapies
    Cilebrex (celecoxib) - NSAID, COX-2
    Vioxx (rofecoxib) - NSAID, COX-2
    Arthro-7 (a natural product by GVL)

NSAID - Nonsteroidal anti-inflammatory drugs
GVL - Gero Vita Laboratories
COX-2 - Cyclooxygenase form that inhibits much lower levels of an important enzyme

ARTHRITIS BOOKS (examples):

Arthritis: What Exercises Work by Dava Sobel and Arthur C. Klein
a spectrum of activity-aerobics (like walking), stretching (like yoga), strengthening (like weights or isometrics).

How to eat away Arthritis by Lauri Aesoph
Based on a simple diet of health-building, restorative foods.

The John Hopkins White Papers on Arthritis by Simeon Margolis and John Flynn

Reverse Your Arthritis Naturally! A report offered by Dr. Julian Whitaker with his Health & Healing subscription.

(Cutting back or eliminating fruits particularly citrus fruits has shown to be of help to some).

10 What your Body's Organs can be telling You or just things to Know

The Skin

According to some authorities in nutrition, the dry scaly skin of psoriasis is produced as a result of too much mucus in our bodies and of nutritional starvation. An excess of mucus is developed in the intestinal tract by the imbalance created by stress and improper eating habits. The excess mucus blocks moisture and nutrients from being absorbed properly by the intestines, causing the body to use alternative supplies (waste products, toxins, poisons). The consequence is an imbalance on an already overtaxed system, creating side-effects such as psoriasis as well as a variety of other diseases.

Following, is an explanation of dry skin and its treatment, written by Elizabeth Burda Venchuk, R.Ph. and published by the National Psoriasis Foundation:

Simple Dry Skin and its Treatment

The skin is sometimes referred to as the largest organ of the human body. Yes, it is an organ. It is a complex structure and carries out functions of its own. The most important function of the skin is to protect our internal organs from infection. The top layer of skin is called the epidermis. It is composed of three layers, the stratum corneum, the stratum lucidum and the stratum granulosum. The latter two layers function to generate skin cells. The stratum corneum is the layer which most of us see. It is the topmost layer of skin, also known as the barrier layer. This layer helps to prevent water loss from the underlying tissues.

The most common condition affecting the skin is dry or chapped skin. Dry skin in itself is not a life threatening condition. However, it produces itching and sometimes pain and inflammation, which in turn can lead to infection. Dry skin is not due to lack of oils, as most of us think, but is due to a lack of water or inadequate hydration. In normal skin, the stratum corneum should contain about 10% water A number of factors can decrease normal skin hydration, and one of the most important is relative humidity. When the stratum corneum has 10% water content, which occurs at about 60% relative humidity, the keratin will soften. The greater the humidity, the softer the skin, and vice versa. Thus in the cold winter months when the humidity is low, dry skin is most prevalent. Age can also affect the skin. As individuals get older, the epidermal skin layer becomes thinner and thus the ability to retain moisture decreases. Excessive bathing (more than once every one to two days) can also lead to dry skin primarily because soaps and detergents can cause damage to the stratum corneum's cells.

The treatment of dry skin is to raise the stratum corneum moisture level. Water is what the skin needs, but simply adding water is not practical if the stratum corneum cannot retain it. If the skin is not covered immediately with petrolatum or a plastic covering, it will dehydrate quickly. There are several ways to treat dry skin. These are:

1. to lubricate the skin
2. to moisturize the skin
3. to chemically soften the keratin layer

A lubricant is defined as any substance that lessens friction. Lubricants do not actually increase the moisture level of the stratum corneum. They do, however, make the skin feel smooth. And if the skin is smooth to the touch, the individual feels good. The most common lubricants used are bath oils. These are generally diluted with bath water and therefore are present in low concentrations. Bath oils are not very effective treating dry skin when used this way. However, they are effective when applied as wet compresses directly to the skin or as a rubdown. For use as a rubdown, mix one teaspoonful of bath oil per 1/4 cup of warm water. Bath oils can also be more effective if applied to the skin immediately after bathing.

The second approach to treating dry skin is the use of moisturizing agents. The most common agents used are humectants and occlusives. Glycerin and propylene glycol are the most widely used humectants. Humectants act by absorbing water from the atmosphere and therefore serve as a reservoir for the stratum corneum. But these products are only useful when the air is saturated with moisture (when relative humidity is high) and when humidity is high, the incidence of dry skin is low. Even so, products containing 20-50% diluted glycerin are still effective in treating dry skin, because glycerin has another mechanism of action. Glycerin speeds up the rate of moisture diffusion from the dermis up to the surface of the skin and also holds this water in close contact with the stratum corneum. Glycerin also acts as a lubricant, making the skin feel better However, undiluted or pure glycerin should not be used to treat dry skin because it can have a dehydrating effect.

Occlusive agents on the other hand are hydrophobic, meaning water-hating. These agents act by providing a barrier on the surface and thus preventing moisture evaporation from the underlying skin. Occlusive agents are also referred to as emollients and include petrolatum, lanolin, silicones and mineral oil. When treating dry skin with occlusives, soak the area in tepid water for 5-10 minutes and then apply the agent immediately to the skin. Petrolatum is the most effective of the occlusives. It should not be applied to open wounds or infected skin as it may cause further inflammation.

Mineral oil is not as occlusive and silicones are less effective. Lanolin is derived from sheep wool. In susceptible individuals, it can cause an allergic reaction and therefore is not frequently used. Most patients have an aversion to occlusives because of their greasiness and difficulty in spreading, so these products have been reformulated and diluted to form emulsions, commonly referred to as creams and lotions. Emulsions can be oil-in-water or water-in-oil depending on the concentration of the ingredients. Emulsions are less effective but they are more acceptable.

Finally we can soften the keratin layer by using chemical agents. Urea, lactic acid and allontoin are some agents used. Urea has the advantage of being less greasy and also is capable of removing thick crusted and scaly skin such as on the bottom of the feet. Urea in concentrations of 10% is used to treat simple dry skin while 20-30% concentrations are used to treat crusted and scaly dry skin. Some people are sensitive to urea and it can produce a stinging or burning effect on initial application. Lactic acid is used in concentrations of 2-5% to treat dry skin. It is also available in a 12% concentration, in Lac-Hydrin lotion, which is a prescription only product in the USA and an OTC product in Canada. Allontoin has been used in 0.5-2.0% concentrations. It is less effective than urea but has proven to be safer for individuals who are sensitive to other products. It is also considered safe for infants and children.

Elliott Douglas Derzaph

Selection of the most appropriate product largely depends on patient acceptance. Gels or oil-in-water emulsions are more acceptable for use on hands, feet, face or skin folds where greasy products are unacceptable. We realize the information contained in this article is technical. We suggest that you take the article and any questions to your dermatologist for discussion.

(National Psoriasis Foundation®, The RX Allstates Pharmacy Service Digest, "Simple Dry Skin and its Treatment," 1986, 6600 SW 92nd Ave., Suite 300, Portland, OR 97223. Reprinted by permission)

The Human Body Series by Torstar Books, 1984, includes an excellent, highly detailed book on the skin titled: Skin: The Human Fabric. It is available in most libraries.

The Colon

The colon is considered by many doctors to be the origin of many diseases, including psoriasis. The colon is a hollow, tube-like organ, extending from the cecum, where the small intestine empties undigested food, down to the rectum, a distance of approximately five to six feet. The walls of the colon have several layers of muscular tissue which expand and contract propelling the contents of the digestive tract slowly from cecum to rectum. The inner lining contains sensitive nerves and glands. The glands aid in the final stages of digestion and assimilation of food - especially minerals and water - and in eliminating body wastes from the system.

When an individual is under stress, the digestive tract may be affected. In fact, nearly 50% of all stress affects the digestive tract. When under stress, the muscular contractions of the colon are not able to sweep the packed and hardened fecal matter along the digestive canal, resulting in stasis, the beginning of constipation.

When a person is constipated, the walls of the colon are generally packed or lined with accumulated fecal matter from many months or years of intestinal cramming. Most people have a colon that might be compared to a water pipe which is partly obstructed by mineral deposits and corrosion. Thus, you can imagine why the colon can neither absorb nor eliminate properly for most people. Foods remain undigested. Tablets and capsules are seen by colon therapists passing through entirely whole. Wastes from the blood arrive at the inner wall of the colon to be absorbed through the wall of the intestine - but they cannot pass this area crammed with hardened fecal matter - so they are reabsorbed into the body. Add to this, the toxins resulting from the fermentation and putrefaction of undigested food and you can see that the poisons that the body is trying unsuccessfully to get rid of can be constantly bathing delicate body cells. The result: "unwellness" and illness. It has been stated that constipation is the most common denominator in diseases.

Most adults probably have an instinctive dislike for their own waste products. This may explain why physicians, in general, are often so remiss in examining their patients' feces, and why so many bowel conditions are not diagnosed and consequently neglected.

Probably more diseases and problems originate in this area of the body than any other. Toxic substances, including gases, are formed from undigested proteins and other foods. A group of physicians in England reported that "Death begins in the colon." In the Chapter on "A Healthy Colon" you will learn how to alleviate some of the problems of the colon.

Other Organs

Knowing how your body works is important so that you understand how your organs can be affected by your particular ailment. Listed here are several organs that can play a part in skin problems, specifically psoriasis. The excerpts that follow are taken from *Gray's Anatomy* and the *Medical Dictionary for the Non-professional* (except for the information on the adrenal glands).

> **Adrenal glands** - One description of this gland is that it is sends energy to the skin, kidneys and up and down the spine. The pair of endocrine glands secrete hormones directly into the bloodstream. Each of the adrenal glands has different functions. The outer region secretes aldosterone which inhibits the amount of sodium excreted in the urine, maintaining blood volume and blood pressure. The inner region secretes the hormones corticosteroid which effects the body's metabolism, the way in which energy is stored and food is used and hydrocortisone helps the body recover from stress, and chemicals the blood secretes. Also, it is part of the sympathetic nervous system, the body's first line of response and defense against physical and emotional stresses.
>
> The adrenal gland may be a good example to try using direct communication between your consciously verbally stating a message to an organ of your own body. You can find many books in the market place where research with doctors found that mind/body

communication have assisted in the health of an individual. You clearly tell the organ often exactly what its job is to be part of a healthy system.

Blood system - From the heart, the pure blood is carried through various arterial branches to all parts of the body. In its passage through the capillaries the blood gives up to the tissues the materials necessary for their growth and nourishment, and at the same time receives from the tissues the waste products resulting from their metabolism, and in doing so becomes changed from pure blood into impure blood and is returned to the heart or the liver.

Colon - The colon is divided into four parts - the ascending, transverse, descending and the sigmoid flexure. *(see Chapter 17: "A Healthy Colon: Internal Washing Cleanses the Body".)*

Digestive system - The apparatus for the digestion and absorption of food consists of the alimentary canal and of certain accessory organs. The alimentary canal is a musculo-membranous tube, about thirty feet in length, extending from the mouth to the anus, and lined throughout its entire extent by mucus membrane. Also, the system secretes enzymes used in the digestion of foods.

Gallbladder - It is the reservoir for bile. Bile is discharged into the upper part of the digestive tract where it breaks down fats, preparing them further for digestion.

Small intestine - A tube about 20 to 24 feet in length which terminates at the large intestine. This tube is the longest span of the digestive tract. It is a major site of food digestion and absorption of nutrients.

Large intestine - It is about five feet in length and stops at the anus. Part of the digestive system which includes the cecum, appendix, ascending colon, transverse colon, descending colon and the rectum.

Kidney - Organs that filter wastes from the blood and excrete them and water in urine and help to regulate the water, electrolyte, and pH balance of the body. The function of the kidney is controlled by hormones.

Liver - The liver is the largest, and one of the most complex, organs of the body. It is supplied with oxygenated blood and nutrients from the stomach and intestines. The liver has numerous functions: it is a site of protein, carbohydrate, and fat metabolism; it helps regulate the level of blood sugar; it secretes bile, which is stored in the gallbladder before its release into the intestinal tract; it detoxifies poisonous substances; and it breaks down worn out red blood cells.

Lymphatic system - The lymphatic or absorbent glands possess the property of absorbing certain materials from the tissues and conveying them into the circulation. Lymph is a thin fluid that bathes the tissues of the body and enters the blood system.

Some doctors in the U.S. have found that disease is caused by a lack of oxygen at the cell level. One can learn to activate your Lymphatic System which pulls out dead cells and toxins in every part of your body, so the body can be free of disease. We can enhance our system which removes dead cells and allows the blood to bring fresh oxygen, a necessity in speeding up any healing. The Lymphatic System is easily activated basically by being active, deep breathing, bouncing, stroking and compressing tissues.

Pancreas - It excretes several digestive enzymes. Also, it secretes the hormones insulin and glucagon into the bloodstream.

Skin - The skin is the outer covering and the largest organ of the body. It is the principal seat of the sense of touch. It protects the body from injury and invasion by microorganisms, helps (through hair follicles and sweat glands) to maintain body temperature, serves as a sensory network, lubricates and waterproofs the exterior, and serves as an organ of excretion. The skin consists of two layers, which contains nerve endings, hair follicles, glands, lymph vessels, and blood vessels.

Spleen - Part of the lymphatic system produces cells involved in immune responses, it also stores blood and produces red blood cells before birth.

Stomach - The principal organ of digestion that receives partly digested food. In the stomach the food is mixed with the secretions of the gastric glands, chiefly hydrochloric acid and the enzyme, pepsin.

The Cells

At a cellular level, a lesion appears to the body as a wound repair and the activated T-cells make skin cells behave as if there is a wound. The cells reproduce quickly to repair what it thinks is a wound and cause the skin to thicken creating scaly lesions.

T-cells are part of the body's natural defense system to repair damage to it. It has become clear that activated T-cells are driving the disorder called psoriasis according to all the new research being done. The research hasn't shown the trigger yet which could be from the environment, bacterial, an antigen or a viral infection. Normally T-cells do their job then they stop so why do people with psoriasis have T-cells that seem to stay turned on! Genetic research has been looking into this for a few years now.

11 Unleashing the Natural Physician inside: Acupuncture and Chiropractic

Acupuncture

Acupuncture is a medical procedure in which very thin needles are inserted into the skin at specific points in an attempt to cure physical ailments. Acupuncture can be used in conjunction with acupressure and herbs. The goal of acupuncture is to assist the body to function at its optimum, facilitating self-healing.

Presently, an acupuncturist is one of the few types of medical professionals who looks at the "whole system." They become involved with the patient to get a picture of both the physical and the non-physical. The acupuncturist tries to connect emotions and intellect with physical problems. Insights are drawn from what you eat, how you think and feel, inside and out; and by comparing your current level of bodily functions with their optimum level. Acupuncturists may be the most health oriented group in our society. (The approach of the acupuncturist reminds me of, Dr. Leboldus, a family doctor who saw me as a child. He always inquired as to how I felt and how the rest of my life was going while taking care of whatever specific problem was the cause of the visit.)

Dr. Fred Siciliano, a licensed acupuncturist and medicinal herb specialist, practicing Holistic Medicine in Ventura, California, gave me a pamphlet which included the following information.

What is Acupuncture?

Acupuncture is the insertion of tiny needles at specific points or sites on the body surface for therapeutic and medical purposes. This technique regulates physiological functions, stimulates vitality and reduces pain.

Acupuncture is often accompanied by finger-pressure treatment known as "Acupressure" and by heat therapy called "Moxa." These methods enhance the Acupuncture effect.

Elliott Douglas Derzaph

Acupuncture was discovered in China more than 4,000 years ago. It is currently practiced in China, Japan, South East Asia, Sri Lanka, India, Russia, France, Germany, England, Australia and many other places. The World Health Organization endorses the use of Acupuncture for a wide variety of physical conditions.

How Does Acupuncture Work?

Acupuncture has four main theories of operation:

1. Different Acupuncture points stimulate the release of natural substances or chemicals that the body normally produces and requires to function properly.

2. The nervous system pathways are stimulated so that specific organs or organ functions are affected by this stimulation.

3. The body's own, naturally produced, pain relieving substances are stimulated and released. These substances are called "endorphins."

4. Acupuncture stimulates, regulates or normalizes the body's "bio-electrical" current, also called "Chi" or "Vital Energy." This current oversees all body functions and is measurable by special equipment.

What will Acupuncture do for you?

- Reduce short term (acute) or long term (chronic) pain and stimulate your body's own self-healing mechanisms.

- Stimulate individual organ functions, such as: heighten the resistance of the body, improve the metabolism, increase circulatory performance, etc.

- Strengthen your nervous system, encourage the release of stress, and promote a sense of inner calm.

- Assist in the treatment of many internal conditions, such as infection, arthritis, menstrual disorders, etc., when combined with prescribed herbal medicine, nutritional programs, physician's medication and treatment.

- Co-ordinate the interrelating functions of the various organ systems. How these systems work together is just as important, as the individual health of each one.

- Help the body to better assimilate nutrients from foods, vitamins and herbs, etc.

- Encourage the release of physical and emotional trauma due to injury, accident or stress. Unreleased trauma is a major obstacle to good health.

(© Fred Siciliano O.M.D., L.Ac., M.H., Licensed Acupuncturist & Medicinal Herb Specialist. Reprinted by permission.)

My personal experience is that acupuncture has been beneficial in many areas of health. Specific treatments and herbs have been quite successful in alleviating my psoriasis symptoms at times while not having any effect at other times. I have never had any negative side effect from any acupuncture treatment.

Chiropractic
The Edgar Cayce Phenomenon
as it relates to
Psoriasis and Eczema

The following article was written by Dr. John O.A. Pagano, who is a lecturer for the Association for Research and Enlightenment (A.R.E.), the organization that collects, catalogues and disseminates the readings of Edgar Cayce. Dr. Pagano practices chiropractic in Englewood Cliffs, New Jersey.

On March 18, 1877, a man by the name of Edgar Cayce was born on a farm near Hopkinsville, Kentucky. He was born of simple American Heritage and had an extremely limited education even according to the standards of his day. Early in his life, however, he demonstrated astonishing mental perceptions that later made people refer to him as a "prophet in his own time." He made use of his ability especially working with doctors in matters of health, for a period of 45 years before he died at Virginia Beach, Virginia in 1945 at the age of 67.

He was able to diagnose and suggest remedies for the sick and ailing that not only proved to be incredibly accurate as far as the anatomy, physiology and pathology was involved on a particular individual, but his recommendations, if followed through, more often than not brought about considerable relief if not a complete cure, of whatever it was that was ailing the patient.

Among the many health problems covered was that of psoriasis. There are two volumes available on the subject based on the Cayce discourses. I found it quite fascinating to learn that psoriasis, according to Cayce, has its origin not in the skin, but in the intestinal tract! He described it as the body's attempt to throw off accumulated toxins (poisons) through the skin rather than through the primary channels of elimination; namely bowels and kidneys. He described the cause in many cases as being due to the presence of thin or flattened intestinal walls, especially in the first section of the small intestines that allowed these toxins to "seep" through the walls of the intestines which are then picked up by the lymphatic system and subsequently "dumped" as it were, into the blood circulatory system. From there the blood normally courses through the liver and kidneys for purification - but sooner or later, the toxic accumulation becomes excessive, too much for the liver and kidneys to handle. The skin then goes into action and helps eliminate these toxins through the sweat glands.

Although the thinning of the intestinal walls were described as the root cause in several cases he diagnosed, it was not the only cause. There is, however, one factor that is consistent with all psoriasis and eczema cases, that the toxic accumulations override the body's ability to adequately discharge them.

That, in its simplest terms, is the Cayce theory of the cause of psoriasis; and strange as it may seem, the same applies to eczema.

Sounds reasonable to me! Why not? It's better than any other theory I've ever heard about psoriasis. Naturally, the next question is - can it be proven? The concept, in theory at least, was not that impossible to fathom. Little did I know that I would spend the greater part of my professional career proving the theory was valid.

What made it valid? Simple - by the results attained on a great many patients! I aspire to the philosophy that if you do the wrong thing you can never get the right result; whereas, if you do the right thing, you cannot get a wrong result. Now, after many years of practical experience with psoriasis and eczema patients, I say without reservation that Cayce was right - right indeed!

Dr. Pagano looks upon Edgar Cayce Reading #2455-2 as the Great Gift to every psoriasis sufferer: When asked if there was an absolute cure for psoriasis, Cayce answered - "Most of the cure is found in Diet. There is a cure. It requires patience, persistence, and Right Thinking also."

Psoriasis: The Struggle and the Triumph
A Healthy Transformation for Everyone Living with Psoriasis

The following is excerpted from an article by Dr. John Pagano, which appeared in the August 1987 issue of *Venture Inward*, published by the Edgar Cayce Foundation.

Chiropractic: Beyond Backaches

Maintaining the integrity of the human spine by manual manipulation rings loud and clear as a major health measure throughout the Cayce readings.

During my college years, I can recall being captivated by the works of Cayce, particularly as they pertain to spinal adjustments. His readings on the subject reinforced my beliefs about the efficacy of adjusting the spine for the restoration and preservation of health, with one added benefit: they explained why adjustments of the spine were vitally important.

From those early days to the present, a span of 35 years, I have experienced and witnessed results from a spinal manipulation that still puts me in awe of the principle. Far from being a technique capable only of relieving backache, spinal adjustments, according to Cayce, as well as chiropractic theory, can affect the various organs of the viscera that ordinarily are not associated in therapy with the cause of disease. The Cayce works not only emphasize the importance of looking to the spine for the cause of disease but specifically name the vertebrae involved.

As an example, in cases of psoriasis and eczema, two widely spread skin diseases, Cayce pinpoints the segments of the spine to be adjusted as the 6th and 7th dorsal with combined adjusting of the 3rd cervical, 9th dorsal and 4th lumbar.

Another question the readings clarify in regard to chiropractic philosophy is the frequent use of the term "subluxation." Subluxation, the term to describe a vertabra out of its proper alignment with the vertebra above and below it, is a chiropractic term. It is the anatomical/physiological principle upon which his profession rests. Until recently, the term subluxation was not only ignored by the medical fraternity but labeled non-existent Now, however, as is evidenced by US Government Medicare and Medicaid guide-lines, the subluxation not only is recognized as a primary cause of disease, but it is mandatory that it, as well as the type, be specifically listed on all forms.

The Cayce readings quite often used the term "subluxated" vertebrae when referring to causes of disease.

As a matter of fact, one particular Cayce Reading (#4001) clearly states that one subluxation could be the cause of some psoriasis cases because of the effect it could have on the integrity of the intestinal walls leading to an eventual breakdown of these walls allowing the seepage of toxic elements to take place. In modem day parlance this is referred to as "The Leaky Gut Syndrome." Instead of subluxation, the osteopathic profession refers to this shift in articular facets as a "spinal lesion." In essence, they are the same and the principle of treatment is the same: align the vertebrae by manual manipulation. The purpose is not only to relieve the irritation developed at the site of misalignment, even though slight, at the articulations, but to release the nerve energy flowing from the central nervous system, through the intervertebral foramen that has been altered by the subluxated vertebrae.

Then, according to chiropractic as well as Cayce philosophy, the body is capable of healing itself in many cases. This, in itself follows a reading (1967-1) often quoted in Cayce literature when discussing the true force in healing:

> "Know that all strength, all healing of every nature is the changing of the vibrations from within - the attuning of the Divine within the living tissue of a body to Creative Energies. This alone is healing. Whether it is accomplished by the use of drugs, the knife or what not, it is the attuning of the atomic structure of the living cellular force to its spiritual heritage."

To deny or refuse to believe that a spinal subluxation can adversely affect the internal organs of the viscera, glands or special senses, and that the correction of this condition by spinal manipulation may restore them to normal function is to ignore the very precepts of neuro-physiological function.

We know that every organ of the body depends upon an adequate flow of nerve impulses to function normally. If for one reason or another, that nerve impulse is altered, changed or blocked, the end organ it supplies will suffer the consequences and eventually break down on a cellular level. This may be likened to a short circuit in a wiring system.

One of the major causes of that alteration of nerve impulses is pressure placed on the nerve root as is emanates from the opening between each spinal segment. The affected organ depends upon the segment involved very much like a switchboard Spinal subluxations *or lesions are a primary cause of that pressure on the nerve root. The principle of chiropractic and osteopathic therapy is that properly applied manual manipulation or adjustment can relieve the pressure on the nerve root, thus restoring the normal flow of neurological impulses, which subsequently restores the depleted end organ to its normal physiological function.*

The doctor doesn't heal anything, he removes blockages to allow the body to heal itself.

The basic Cayce concept of healing - that the healing comes from within, and the doctor only assists - was recognized nearly 2,500 years ago by Hippocrates, the Father of Medicine, when he courageously stated: "The gods are the real physicians, although people do not think so." By "gods" he meant nature and its mysterious forces, power and laws.

(© Dr. John O.A. Pagano, reprinted by permission.)

Dr. Pagano's book, HEALING PSORIASIS: *The Natural Alternative,* was voted "Best Book of the Year" in the category of Health by the North American Bookdealers Exchange (N.A.B.E.) for 1991. The book is available from The Pagano Organization, Inc., 35 Hudson Terrace, Box 1215, Englewood Cliffs, New Jersey 07632, Telephone: 201-947-4001, 800-919-4001. The cost is $24.95, plus $4.00 shipping & handling (New Jersey residents add $1.50 sales tax).

It is very common to hear the so called "Old Guard of Medicine" fighting to restrict new players into the realm of health care. This occurs even after the new health service is legally, ethically and professionally approved by our country's legitimate authorities.

A few years ago, I came across a book that might be of interest. Dr. Karl V. Holmquist, a chiropractor, wrote *Home Chiropractic Handbook,* to help simplify the understanding of chiropractic principles. Dr. Holmquist's intention is to help people to assist in the process of being healthy. He does not intend for his book to replace doctors or chiropractors.

Dr. Holmquist gives a number of examples and thorough explanations of the world of a chiropractor in his book.

Chiropractic is a philosophy, science and art dedicated to restoring normal nerve transmission in the body and further, to maintain that normality.

Elliott Douglas Derzaph

Health in the body is directly related to normal nerve function from brain cell to tissue cell. Gray's Anatomy, which is considered a bible of anatomy among the health professions, defines the brain and spinal cord as the central nerve system or the master controlling system. We need only consider who created the human brain, and we know by its magnificent construction that it is the finest computer ever 'built'. The computer (brain and spinal cord) simply "tells" the body what to do through its "message transmitters" (nerves.) The brain is connected to every cell of the body through the intricate message system. To prove this to yourself just wiggle one hair on your arm. This will stimulate that single hair follicle, relaying a message over nerves, communicating back to your brain. Every cell in every organ of the body is also "told what to do" by the brain through the nerve system. Although you are not conscious of what your internal body parts are doing or even should be doing, the subconscious centers of your brain are sending messages over the nerves and telling every organ and cell what to do and further, coordinating every organ and cell into harmony. Understanding and maintaining the relationship is the key to health through chiropractic. That is, the brain must coordinate messages to every cell (all parts) so that these parts can function normally. If there is interruption in the message due to misaligned vertebrae that put pressure on the spinal cord or spinal nerves, then the body part that receives those nerve messages stops functioning normally and disease may begin to develop.

Direct pressure on the spinal cord caused by a misaligned atlas can cut nerve transmission (communication) on entire nerve trackways (millions of nerve fibers) all at once, resulting in disease in the body.

To give you an idea of just how complex one system is, we shall briefly discuss the nerve system. In studying anatomy, you will discover that within a system there is a system. For example, there is the spinal nerve system consisting of thirty-one paired spinal nerves, and there is a cranial nerve system consisting of twelve paired cranial nerves dropping directly from the cranial vault. These two nerve systems are connected by a sympathetic and parasympathetic system which have the job of speeding up or slowing down nerve impulses between the spinal nerves and cranial nerves. Further, all of these nerve systems are coordinated and regulated by the master system, the brain and spinal cord.

Psoriasis: The Struggle and the Triumph
A Healthy Transformation for Everyone Living with Psoriasis

When you consider the fact that a misaligned vertebra impairs the communication of the brain and spinal cord, with various end organs, resulting in many types of disease. Therefore, vertebral misalignments cause disease as well as pain, disc deterioration and loss of mobility in the spine. However if vertebrae are properly aligned, they actually protect the spinal cord and insure good health throughout the body.

A subluxated (misaligned) vertebra interferes with normal nerve transmission. It should be distinctly clear at this point that a misaligned vertebra can drastically cut down communication of the brain with any body part and thereby cause malfunction and disease.

It takes the right direction, applying pressure to a point of tension, providing sufficient force with speed, to set the vertebra in motion and reestablish its normal position.

Chiropractic care was originally developed with the idea of providing health maintenance in an intelligent manner.

Chiropractic spinal correcting is a way to bring the entire body into a healthy state. Once the body is brought into a healthy state, then we should maintain that health by continual upkeep, which includes spinal correcting throughout one's life.

Every doctor who has diligently studied the anatomy and physiology of the human body is humbled by its magnificence in construction and performance.

There are no doctors, no scientists, no human beings that have ever healed anything. None of them even know what life is! How could they heal anything! The one power that created the body heals the body. The job of doctors would simply be to get the parts in order so that the healing life power can express properly through the form.

If you can accept, through logical reasoning, that it is not the doctor that does the healing but the power within the body which built the body that does the healing, then you are on the right track to solving health problems.

It is now postulated by modern medical science that 80 to 90 percent of all disease is caused by stress.

(© 1985 *Home Chiropractic Handbook* by Karl V. Holmquist D.C. One 8 Incorporated, P.O. Box 2075, Forks, WA 98331. Reprinted by permission.)

Dr. Velma Scott is a friend and chiropractor. In studying diseases, and in particular, psoriasis, she found three factors which have a significant effect on a person's health.

The first, is consistently eating a nutritionally sound diet, to which should be added vitamins, minerals and specific herbs. The second, is the continual maintenance of the spine by manipulation. The manipulation can be done by someone such as a chiropractor, with skilled hands; or by the individual himself, using specific daily exercises that perpetuate fluidity of the spine. Third, to these we must add attitude, if one does not already have a happy, positive attitude, it must be cultivated.

I recently visited with Dr. Velma Scott. We discussed her recent, one-month trip to China. A few weeks after our visit she mailed me a note describing her exhilaration after a camping trip with her son in a national park in Texas. Dr. Scott had also just celebrated her 86th birthday.

A fluid or flexible spine accompanied by good posture has been hailed for centuries in many Far East countries as a necessity for good health. The most helpful activity I have ever found for keeping the spine healthy is yoga. My personal preference is Kundalini Yoga. It is interesting to note that a fair percentage of yogis I have met are chiropractors.

I recommend chiropractic treatment to put your spine in proper alignment. Once aligned you should start yoga or some other form of movement which will perpetuate flexibility of the spine. Maintaining proper posture should be part of your daily regiment for maintaining a healthy spine.

12 New and Traditional Medications/Drugs

Most over-the-counter (OTC) drugs and prescription drugs have side-effects; and every patient should clearly understand the potentially dangerous nature of these side-effects. In a (4/14/92) documentary on a public access television station it was stated that "15,000 people die from side-effects of drugs in the U.S. each year."

Drugs are (frequently) synthetically created chemical reproductions of one or more natural products. Companies today manufacture a whole spectrum of synthetic substances, from ice (chemical cold packs) to rare drugs created from plants found only in the jungles of the Amazon.

Chemical substances are not bad in and of themselves. In fact, the brain itself produces thousands of neurochemicals. The difference is that drugs assault the whole brain while the brain's own neurochemicals release in a very specific location and do not influence any other part, thereby, producing the needed result without side-effects. The wise use of drugs should be the goal of any human wishing sound and healthy results.

The following article appeared in the Fall 1991 edition of the Canadian Psoriasis Foundation (C.P.F.) newsletter, under the heading of "New Products On the Market:"

"Psori-aid" capsules

In a study conducted by Dr. Allan Lassus (Department of Dermatology, University Central Hospital, Helsinki, Finland), psoriasis sufferers were given **Psori-aid** *capsules, a Swedish preparation imported by Scandinavian Pharmaceuticals of Pennsylvania, USA, in which the natural active ingredient is a specific polyunsaturated ethyl ester lipid, easily metabolized. No inflammatory agents were released by those in the study group, symptoms decreased and cell function returned to normal, and when 'Psori-aid' cream was also used, results were even more pronounced. 'Psori-aid' shampoo decreased itchy scalp discomfort.*

Even the unaffected skin of people with psoriasis is drier than normal and 'SuperGlandin Day and Night Cream' relieves that irritation because it contains essential gamma linolenic acid (GLA.)

Elliott Douglas Derzaph

> *'Psori-aid' is now available in Canadian health food stores. For further information call Sisu Enterprises (1-800-663-4163/Canada.)*

(© 1991, Canadian Psoriasis Foundation (C.P.F.) from the C.P.F. Newsletter, Volume 7, Number 1, Fall 1991. Reprinted by permission.)

(Update: 'Psori-aid' is now called 'X-ORI'. They offer a shampoo and cream along with the capsules - 60 count for $24. In the U.S. information can be received by sending a SASE to Scandinavian Natural Health & Beauty Products, Inc., 13 N. 7th St., Perkasie, PA 18944

Dr. Karl V. Holmquist, in his Home Chiropractic Handbook, wrote about the use of drugs:

> *People are led to believe when they take a drug such as aspirin, the drug is transmitted only to that part of the body intended to receive it. Television commercials for aspirin show a special tube from the stomach to the brain. This is misleading and absolutely not true! Every drug that is either swallowed by mouth or injected by needle is absorbed into the bloodstream and pumped to every organ, all tissue and ultimately to every cell of the body! Further, the drug may act upon some part or system of the body in a pernicious manner and as a result side effects are often experienced.*
>
> *It should be known that your body makes every antibody, every drug and every chemical automatically in the exact quantity and perfect quality required for your unique individual needs.*
>
> *It should be noted that medical crisis therapy may be required if the body has not been maintained in health and if parts of the body have seriously deteriorated. However, drugs should be very carefully and discriminately prescribed by medical doctors only. Surgery to remove any organ should be considered only as a very last resort.*

Here are some of the questions you may want to ask your doctor after he prescribes drugs for you and your pharmacist before he has filled the prescription.

- What is the name of the medication (both brand name and generic)?

- What should I know about this drug?

- Will it interact with other drugs I may be taking?

- Will it interact with any foods I eat?

- Will it interact with any therapies or treatment I am undergoing?

- How will I know if it's working?

- What are the side-effects of this drug?

- How long should I wait before reporting to my doctor if there is no change in my symptoms?

Refer to the chapter on - Appendix - References and Product Resources, the subsection "Prescription Drug Resources" for books and suppliers of drugs which would be used in the treatment of psoriasis.

Elliott Douglas Derzaph

13 European remedy: GH3?

Gerovital H3 (GH3) was developed in Romania by Dr. Ana Aslan and has been used since 1956 for the treatment of chronic degenerative diseases. The product was named Gerovital to stress its revitalizing action in advanced age. H3 is used as a symbol for the vitamin-like action of the product.

GH3's basic ingredients are procaine, sulphur, potassium and sodium, of which procaine is the active ingredient. Many research studies carried out in Romania and abroad are reported to have confirmed the superiority of Gerovital H3 over all other solutions of procaine. The GH3 treatment depends on the patient's biological age and pathology.

The following excerpts are from the book GH3: Will It Keep You Younger Longer, by Herbert Bailey:

> *Procaine is a synthetic combination of two substances naturally occurring in the body. Inside the body procaine breaks down into its original components. PABA (para-aminobenzoic acid) and DEAE (diethylaminoethanol). They perform certain jobs in the brain, nerve tissue and various other organs.*
>
> *The difference between procaine and GH3 is that GH3 is stable for at least two years. The use of a preservative and antioxidant preserve the life of the procaine molecule in the body Ordinary procaine is rapidly destroyed when it enters the bloodstream. GH3, with its buffer, has an acid balance and is intact in the body after six hours, giving it much longer to react on the brain and nervous centers.*
>
> *As GH3 breaks down, it releases its two constituents PABA and DEAE. They, too, have an important role before they are metabolized. PABA stimulates the "good" intestinal flora to produce such needed vitamins as folic acid and vitamins K and B1 (thiamine.) DEAE participates in the making of choline and acetylcholine, vital factors in the body (liver and spleen), brain and nerve synapses.*

(GH3: *Will It Keep You Younger Longer*, by Herbert Bailey, copyright 1977-1980. Reprinted by permission of Bantam Books.)

The effectiveness of the tissue regenerating action of Gerovital H3 is especially evident on the skin and extraskeleton (outside part of the 206 bones in our body that make up the skeleton) where it produces a rejuvenating appearance.

GH3 is used in Romania, Eastern Europe, Europe, South America and North America (including the U.S.). GH3's usage and acceptance follows the above order.

GH3 treatment is a combination of tablets and injections. You start by administering intramuscular injections of one ampoule three times a week, a series of 12 injections in 4 weeks. Then, there is a rest period of two weeks, followed by a period of 12 days in which you take two tablets a day, two to three hours after meals. You then take another rest period of four weeks, then repeat the sequence of 12 injections and 24 tablets. This completes one period of treatment. The number of treatments depends on the individual. Larger doses of the tablets have shown to be almost as effective as the injections.

GH3 is indicated in *trophic* (nutrition related) disorders such as peripheral arteriosclerosis, degenerative rheumatism, dystrophia of the skin, nails and hair, eczema and psoriasis.

I have used GH3 several times as a comprehensive health aid, in the same way that one would use vitamin B12 injections. During the first few times I received injections of GH3, I noticed significant improvements in my psoriasis. Later injections or the use of the pills alone resulted in little or no improvement at all. The factors that may have affected the results in the latter use were: I purchased the GH3 from a different source and was unsure if the product was authentically produced in Romania. I was living alone without the help of another person, placing myself in a very tense situation, requiring acrobatic contortions, to inject the GH3 into my gluteus maximus. The self injections were difficult and stressful and I did not follow the proper treatment schedule and recommended procedure.

GH3 requires further research in controlled environments in testing and production in locations like an European, Canadian or American reputable health organization.

Elliott Douglas Derzaph

14 Nutrition Health options

When a successful salesman/friend talked to me about the products he marketed, he said "you never have to explain quality twice." To me, that philosophy describes how we should look at our health. We should give ourselves quality time, quality activities and quality food, to enhance the health of our body and our mind.

Health, according to Dr. John Harrison, is not an absence of disease. It's a willingness to take responsibility for any disease we choose to give ourselves. I believe that self-responsibility implies a continuing improvement in those things over which we have control. It does not imply we have control over everything.

In USA Weekend, August 21, 1994, an article began: "Meet Jean Carper, health expert, author of *Food - Your Miracle Medicine* and an award-winning T.V. medical correspondent. Starting today, she delivers sensible, scientific advice in 'Eat Smart,' her new monthly column in *USA Weekend.*" In the first paragraph she stated, "You can stay healthy, stave off disease and possibly even reverse illness with what you eat. That's a fact, proved by a constant flow of food/health research."

The following is excerpted from an article published by the National Psoriasis Foundation (N.P.F.):

> Psoriasis is characterized by a too-rapid production of skin cells, and many people are searching for a dietary means of slowing the cell turnover. They may be taken aback to learn that there is one such diet remedy, although it is one in which the cure is worse than the disease. The remedy is called starvation.
>
> Researchers today know that protein controls cell growth. A diet with little or no protein, whether from vegetable or animal sources, will slow the rapid cell growth that characterizes psoriasis.
>
> Physicians have noted that the skin of psoriasis patients will sometimes improve while they are on a weight-loss diet and that weight gain can cause psoriasis to flare or worsen.
>
> Occasionally people have written to say that their psoriasis improved while they were hospitalized from some other cause than skin problems and were being nourished by intravenous feedings. They have asked if something in the solution had a beneficial effect on psoriasis.

Psoriasis: The Struggle and the Triumph
A Healthy Transformation for Everyone Living with Psoriasis

(National Psoriasis Foundation®. Reprinted by permission)

At the 1992 National Psoriasis Conference, Dr. Janet Prystowsky presented a lecture on the topic, "Nutrition and Psoriasis." Basically, she concluded that psoriasis can cause certain nutritional deficiencies. Dr. Prystowsky also stated that psoriasis can affect the body's normal amount of: protein, folate, iron, water and calories; and nutritional supplementation will not remedy psoriasis though they will improve your general health.

All of us recognize that a good diet is mandatory for good health. People with psoriasis who normally are healthy and slender appear to do best in controlling their psoriasis and have the least severe cases.

Some general principles for maintaining good health include:

- Eat healthy

- Eat less (especially after the age of 25)

- Eat all foods in moderation

- Quit eating 2 hours before sleeping and never load up your stomach during the evening hours especially with protein

- Rest/relax 15 minutes before, and 15-30 minutes after, eating, for good digestion

- Breakfast is the most important, and should be the largest meal of the day

- Drink fluids alone or at least 15-30 minutes before or after a meal

- Vary the types of foods eaten

- Do not eat when upset

- Chew well

- Daily food intake should consist of at least 50% vegetables (raw or lightly steamed)

- Remember, it is common to crave whatever foods to which you are allergic.

Elliott Douglas Derzaph

Digestion is the process of converting the food we eat into the fuel needed to support life in our bodies. The better the quality of the fuel, the better the body runs. Digestion takes the greatest amount of energy of all bodily tasks except for physical activity. Knowing digestive times might help determine your eating patterns.

The time it takes for food to pass through the digestive and eliminative systems are as follows:

- The stomach - 1 to 6 hours
- The small intestine - 2 to 9 hours
- The large intestine - 1 to 3 days

The time it takes for various types of food to pass through the digestive and eliminative systems are as follows:

- Fruit - less than 24 hours
- Vegetables - less than 24 hours (but slightly longer than fruits)
- Fish, fowl and grains - more than 1 day but usually less than 2 days
- Dairy products - 2 to 3 days
- Red meat - 3 days

Foods to eat (as fresh as possible):

- Vegetables (in season, especially raw)
- Sprouts
- Garlic (raw or mildly cooked)
- Brazil nuts
- Fruit (in season)
- Fiber
- Whole Grains
- Beans
- Water (8-10 large glasses a day, not cold)

I have observed over the years that when I consume certain products I get a reaction within 24 hours and sometimes within just a few hours. The most noticeable causes have been alcohol, caffeine and sugar. I get a case of severe itching after eating a bowl of anything like ice cream or two to three drinks of alcohol or one cup of caffeinated coffee.

Products to eliminate or greatly reduce are as follows:

- Sugar (refined)
- Fat (most kinds, especially saturated fats and meat fats, such as skins. One theory concluded that psoriasis may result from a faulty utilization of fat).
- Alcohol (dehydrates the body)
- Caffeine
- Drugs (all kinds)
- Dairy products (especially milk, cream, butter)
- Meats (especially red meat)
- Hot Peppers (hot spicy peppers alone or in food, should be avoided except on a modest and irregular basis)

Research found that the individuals who smoked more than 24 cigarettes per day were around twice as likely as non-smokers to develop psoriasis in their lifetime. The risk level decreased proportionate to the number of cigarettes smoked per day. Men who consume three or more alcoholic drinks daily have a greater chance of developing psoriasis than women with the same drinking habits.

If you notice a negative reaction after eating a certain food, it would be sensible to remove it or at least decrease its consumption in your diet. It is a small sacrifice to limit or reduce those things that agitate your system.

Food-combining, allows the individual at each meal to eat foods in a fashion that is the most conducive to optimum digestion. When nutrition and food-combining practices are considered while eating, the body receives the greatest nutritional benefit offered by the food consumed while using the least amount of energy to digest and use the food.

CORRECT FOOD COMBINING

BEST (optimum digestion)

- Eating only one type of food, for example, eating only fruit at a meal

GOOD (good digestion atmosphere)

- Starches with green vegetables
- Proteins with green vegetables

POOR (poor digestion atmosphere)

- Green vegetables with all fruits
- Starches with all fruits; starches with proteins
- Fruits with proteins

(Check your local bookstore for more information on food-combining. One book I suggest is **Food Combining Simplified***, by Dennis Nelson, Nelsons Books.)*

Try to eat fish no more than twice a week and any other type of meat once a week and if possible leave at least 1 day between eating fish and 3 days between eating any other type of meat. If you are going to eat red meat, eat venison or lamb instead of pork and beef. It is normally less or completely free of additives like steroids. Further the animals are not fed their same species as food. Please note that many meat producers do not feed their animals the same species but until those specifics are made known to the consumer, be cautious.

Jackman Gillette, in his book *Psoriasis*: *The Story of a Man who Helped Himself* made note of a simple, yet significant observation after years of personal research on the relationship between his psoriasis and eating.

Gillette wrote about the intense personal journey that brought him to the conclusion that protein starvation will ultimately result in the stoppage of the scaling process and a clearing of psoriatic lesions. He admits it is a challenging process and has side-effects that could be damaging to the rest of the body and worth noting. Extended programs could cause starvation.

Most of us, under normal circumstances, ingest about 75 grams of protein a day - considerably more than the amount required to meet the average adult's protein needs. Nutritionists estimate that only about 22 grams of protein a day is sufficient to supply the needs of the average adult.

The following is a partial list of foods with little or no protein:

- Honey (no protein)
- Apples, cherries, apricots, grapes, cranberries, peaches, pears, pineapple (low protein)
- Carrots, green peppers, radishes, celery, cucumbers, lettuce (low protein)

Dr. Kenneth Thane Walker (writer, psychoanalyst, lecturer), described the essence of good eating habits, "Everything in moderation including moderation." Dr. Walker explained that if we all ate and drank a reasonable amount and consistently varied our diet, we would stay healthy. This also means not consuming an excessive amount of any one item. We would then have an opportunity to eat, without negative consequences, all food products available for human consumption.

We have a tendency to habituate our eating habits, wherein, we consume the same foods over and over on a daily or weekly basis. As a result the body receives more of these items than it needs, resulting in a burden on certain parts of the system. At the same time, such a diet is likely not nutritious.

It is the long term effects of excessive consumption that cause most diseases. If we were to smoke a cigarette or have a drink of alcohol or coffee, just once or twice a week, the effect on our system would be minimal. Unfortunately, we usually don't manage our appetites that well; and unconsciously end up abusing our body to the point of causing significant damage. The damage isn't recognized by most of us until considerable strain is put on our body or a disease is well in place.

Separately packaged frozen fruits and vegetables are quite healthy to eat, because they are fresh, rather than pre-cooked (which destroys nutrients) and do not require additives. Dehydrated food has no additives and is also quite healthy.

Some diet recommendations that will aid psoriasis patients, in particular, are:

- Fruits and vegetables (especially garlic)
- Soups and salads
- Whole grain cereals
- Lecithin (whole grain cereals, wheat germ, lecithin flakes)
- Bran (1-2 teaspoons a day)
- Brewer's Yeast (1 teaspoon a day)
- Honey
- Vinegar
- Wine (red) or grape juice

The basic premise is to get the human body into good working condition, so it can do well in any fight, with any disorder it encounters, such as psoriasis.

Elliott Douglas Derzaph

Drinking juices to replace or supplement a meal will assist in renewing your health. Many juice programs can be found in books or on television. The key is to juice fruits and vegetables when they are as fresh as possible. Juice has the greatest nutritional value when first extracted, so once the juice is made, drink it. Juice has a short life, maybe 4 to 5 days, at most. It's best to get a juice machine that is simple to use and easy to clean. Otherwise, it is too easy to put the machine in the cupboard, until you get around to using it again - which you won't!

Juicing mixture recommended for Psoriasis - celery (½ cup), Swiss chard (1 ½ Tbsp.), and cucumber juice (½ cup) diluted with a little carrot juice (1 cup).

Recommended juices for Psoriasis either homemade or (natural food) store bought juices - Blueberry Juice; Elderberry Juice; Huckleberry Juice and of course Carrot juice. And keep in mind if at all possible avoid carbonated drinks which cause more gas than the body needs.

It is easy to find very reasonably priced, well built and easy to clean machines. Whichever juicer you buy be certain that it transports the juice and pulp to separate and easily detachable or removable containers. Otherwise, you will be doing more cleaning than drinking and, again, the machine may end up in the cupboard.

Wheatgrass juice is a drink with great health benefits, though it may be difficult to acquire a taste for it. Wheatgrass juice works like "Drano" in that it is a natural and powerful cleanser of your system, an effective remover of toxins. It's considered the most effective natural means of aiding or creating a healthy system. You should drink two, three ounce glasses of wheatgrass juice each day.

15 The Natural Approach: Vitamins, Minerals and Herbs

Vitamins

The world of vitamins and minerals offers a variety of recommendations for healing or alleviating the symptoms of psoriasis. The most common recommendations involve megadoses of vitamins including A, B complex, C, D, E, and niacinamide. Also, daily doses of minerals such as iron and zinc are commonly recommended. The herbal world suggests the ingestion of solutions incorporating sarsaparilla, iodine and milk thistle.

Our choices should start with eating the foods with the vitamins and minerals within them and compliment food with natural herbs, then only as a last resort use artificial supplements.

Recent studies including those in 2001 have produced reports demonstrating that massive consumption of any artificially produced products cause havoc to our soma. Our soma works most efficiently when given healthy natural products as in the form of food and water.

Vitamin D

The following is the entire text of the article, "Rx for Psoriasis," by Katie Tyndall, as it appeared in the January 19, 1987 issue of Insight magazine:

Rx for Psoriasis

A form of the sunshine vitamin, vitamin D, has shown itself effective in treating the symptoms of psoriasis, a skin disease characterized by scaly, itchy patches of skin.

In preliminary studies, 14 of psoriasis patients who had not responded to other treatments had a good to excellent reaction to the vitamin therapy, says Dr Michael Holick of Tufts University's Human Nutrition Research Center in Boston.

> *In one, who had had large reddened patches of scaly skin on his legs and feet for 20 years, the patches cleared up immediately after treatment.*
>
> *Doctors know very little about the cause of the disease. They believe it is linked to a disruption in normal cell maturation and growth.*
>
> *Holick and his colleague suspected that the skin of psoriasis patients did not recognize as well as it should a hormone produced by the kidney that stops the proliferation of skin cells. This hormone is a form of vitamin D. Participants in the experiment received the hormone topically and orally.*
>
> *Holick is guardedly optimistic about the results, which he says will have to be confirmed by larger studies before there is any move to make the hormone available as a medication for psoriasis.*

(© 1987, Insight, Katie Tyndall. Reprinted by permission.)

A little over a year later Dr. Holick's research had produced additional insights, concluding that therapies utilizing special hormonal forms of vitamin D are safer and more effective than current treatments such as ultraviolet light and drugs.

To contact Dr. Holick's research team, write to: The Vitamin D Skin and Bone Research Laboratory, Boston University School of Medicine, 80 East Concord St., M-1013, Boston, MA 02118.

The treatment using the product that is chemically similar to vitamin D can now (report 9/95) be used to control cell growth without the redness and skin thinning. Generally, two months of regular treatment can help keep psoriasis away for about six months.

Other Vitamins

Many health magazines and psoriasis organizations have commented on treatments being researched in this area. At U.C.L.A. Medical School researchers are working with *etretin*, a chemical cousin to a synthetic vitamin A derivative known as *etretinate* which can control psoriatic flare-ups but which also causes birth defects. Etretin appears to work well, and may be safer for women of child bearing age.

And, also at the University of California, initial tests showed that psoriasis patients responded well to megadose treatments of fish oil supplements.

Psoriasis sufferers will have to get the products by prescription when available because of the sensitive nature of the vitamin derivatives (products synthetically derived from vitamins by researchers). A medical professional must be involved before treatment is attempted because of the specific megadose requirements of the fish oil supplements.

Calcipotriene, a medicated ointment containing a derivative of vitamin D now has FDA approval and is available by prescription as Dovonex. Drug trials show about 70% of people treated showed marked improvement after eight weeks, with improvement beginning after just two weeks. About 10% treated had complete clearing. Calcipotriene exhibited fewer adverse effects as compared to many prescription ointments; those most frequently observed were: burning, itching or other skin irritation.

There is a lot of controversy about the effective, safe levels of vitamin supplements. There is much discussion about the dangers of taking some vitamins in doses beyond the RDA. Vitamins E, F and K and especially vitamin A are of concern insofar as overdoses or "megadoses" are concerned. Check with a reputable nutritionist or a trained healing arts practitioner, before taking these vitamins. The potentially toxic effects of the overdose could substantially overshadow any potential benefit to your psoriasis.

The *Vitamin Bible* by Earl Mindell says this about psoriasis:

> Though many jokes have been made about this disease, it is no laughing matter to the millions who suffer from it. No one treatment has been found to be totally effective, but the following *has met with much success:*
>
> - *Mindell Vitamin Program (MVP)**
> - *Vitamin A (water soluble), 10,000 IU three times daily, 5 days a week*
> - *B complex, 100 mg. (time release), a.m. and p.m.*
> - *Rose hips vitamin C, 1,000 mg. a.m. and p.m. (this is in addition to the vitamin C called for in the MVP)*
> - *Vitamin E (dry form), 400 IU three times daily*
> - *Increase protein (preferably animal source)*
>
> ** (MVP consists of a high potency multiple vitamin with chelated minerals, preferably time release; vitamin C, 1,000 mg. with bioflavonoids, nutin, hesperifin, and*

Elliott Douglas Derzaph

> *rose hips, time release; and a high potency chelated multiple-mineral supplement.)*

(Reprint permission granted by Warner Books by arrangement with Richard Curtis Associates, Inc.)

Milk Thistle

Milk Thistle: *The Liver Herb* by Christopher Hobbs, is one of two booklets, written about this powerful herb that helps restore the liver's health. Following are excerpts from the booklets.

Hobbs starts with...

> *Medicinal herbs are still used by the majority of the population in the world today for prevention of disease and restoration of wellness. Nine hundred million Chinese people still rely on herbs for a major part of their health care. In the United States, herbs have been largely supplanted by chemical drugs, but their use is becoming increasingly widespread due to the popularity of the health food movement.*
>
> *This booklet will describe one medicinal herb, Silybum marianum, that has attracted much interest in recent years, especially in Europe, where commercial preparations are being manufactured for severe liver diseases like hepatitis and cirrhosis, as well as for liver restoration. Our modern environment is full of stressful chemicals, such as food additives and pesticides. These chemicals need to be processed by the liver so that they can be eliminated by the body. Further, the liver is an important organ in fat digestion which is usually high in the modern diet.*
>
> *One medical doctor I have been in contact with has used Milk Thistle extract in his daily practice for three years. He has had good success (up to fifty percent cure rate) with psoriasis, a disfiguring and uncomfortable skin ailment. He feels that this disease is liver and bowel-related.*

(From *Milk Thistle: The Liver Herb*, by Christopher Hobbs, copyright, Botanica. Reprinted by permission.)

Psoriasis: The Struggle and the Triumph
A Healthy Transformation for Everyone Living with Psoriasis

Dr. Daniel Mowrey, Director of Science, Mountain West Institute of Herbal Science, Salt Lake City, Utah is the author of the second booklet, *New Hope for Liver Health - Milk Thistle.*

A solution for psoriasis

Milk Thistle may also be a valuable and effective treatment for the common skin disorder, psoriasis. This chronic, recurring condition is usually found on the scalp and surfaces of the limbs, especially the elbows, knees and shins.

When the liver can't detoxify substances such as chemicals, high concentrations of endotoxin (poison contained in the cell walls of some bacteria) circulate in the blood stream. Psoriasis is related to these endotoxin concentrations, and to the production of harmful leukotriene cells (those radical oxygen molecules that interfere with normal liver function) which are often found in inflamed livers. Research showing that silymarin or milk thistle treatment slows down the development of these harmful leukotriene cells, may explain empirical reports of improvement in psoriasis patients following milk thistle treatment.

Dermacine

Dermacine "A" is an all natural product produced at the Derma Clinic in Tijuana, Mexico. The clinic states the program is on-going with clearing of 90% and up, after 6 months, in 88% of the patients. When treatment is stopped, symptoms usually recur within 1 to 3 months; then disappear again within 2 months of daily usage. This program requires continual usage, apparently forever. You are on a restricted diet and use Juniper Tar ointment during treatment, and must always keep your skin moist. There are no known side-effects. I purchased this product in Tijuana and used this product for 5 to 6 weeks noticing little change.

Also, from the Derma Clinic is Dermacine (without the "A"), which can only be administered by a doctor, and which is stated to be more effective, in a shorter period, for a longer term before recurrence. You must stay close to the facility for about 3 weeks.

Herbs

I have read of several herbal extracts which purportedly aid in the treatment of psoriasis. A list of them is presented below. After each listing is the name of the individual who suggested the "remedy" if known.

- Burdock seeds homeopathic tincture *(Dian Dincin Buchman)*.
- Juniper wood oil ointment *(Buchman)*.
- Yellow Saffron Tea (*Edgar Cayce*).
- Slippery Elm Bark Powder *(Edgar Cayce)*.
- Camomile Tea *(Cayce)*.
- Sulphur/Rochelle Salts/Cream of Tarter *(Cayce)*. Mix 1 tbsp. of ea., take 1 tsp.; daily, only after 6 osteopathic adjustments.
- Sarsaparilla extract *(Yogi Bhajan)*. Mix 1 bottle of extract with 2 lbs. of honey and 1-1/2 cups hot water; take 2 tbsp. in 8 oz. glass of water daily.
- Vitilikla's is an herbal supplement advertized as natural, safe and side-effect free. The four herbs are from the Brazilian flora.
- GLA (Gamma-linolenic acid) supplement in black-currant oil and evening-primrose oil Natural anti-inflammatories are Ginger and Curcumin.

Acidophilus

Acidophilus is a source of friendly intestinal bacteria. Acidophilus aids the intestines in working at their optimum condition - clean. A steady influx of friendly bacteria is required, since friendly bacteria die within five days. Health food stores offer acidophilus in various forms for storage on the shelf or in the refrigerator.

Colloidal Silver

Colloidal Silver is produced by using distilled water and adding ultra fine particles of positively charged silver using a DC power source. Colloidal Silver is said to rapidly subdue inflamation and promote the healing of lesions. You can drink the solution as well as apply it directly to the skin. I have met people who swear by it for overall health but so far I have not found a psoriasis patient with any success stories.

Shark Cartilage

First, a few definitions:

Angiogenesis - The development of new blood vessels.
Antiangiogenesis - The inhibition of the development of new blood vessels.
Cartilage - A gristle-like supporting connective tissue.
Immunoregulatory - An immune system that is constant.
Mucopolysaccharides - Any of a group of carbohydrates containing an amino sugar and uronic acid (a sugar acid). Mucopoly-saccharides have been found to have an anti-inflammatory effect.

The benefit of the use of cartilage from sharks is a relatively recent discovery in the treatment of psoriasis. Research in this field has been in progress for almost 30 years, in one form or another, both within the U.S. and around the world.

First, shark cartilage is an angiogenesis inhibitor. Although angiogenesis is normally associated with positive body functions such as wound healing and embryonic development, there are many diseases that are caused by, or whose progress is dependent upon, angiogenesis. Psoriasis is associated with angiogenesis and therefore, likely to be controlled by antiangiogenesis, which is promoted by shark cartilage.

Second, the complex carbohydrates in cartilage known as mucopolysaccharides apparently give shark cartilage other therapeutic benefits besides angiogenesis inhibition. It is the mucopolysaccharides that have the immunoregulatory effect, and they also have an anti-inflammatory effect. The mucopolysaccharides chondroitin sulfate A and C have long been known to fight inflammation. It now seems that the naturally occurring form of these compounds in shark cartilage is more effective than synthetically refined mucopolysaccharides.

Patients have been found to respond favorably after six to eight weeks of treatment. The initial oral consumption of nine capsules a day costs about $90 a month. After clearing has occurred, consumption is reduced by about 50%. You can stop consumption, if you choose, and start again when the psoriasis reappears with the same time period required to clear the initial psoriasis.

As in the case with most psoriasis treatments, shark cartilage does not work with everyone, If you do not see improvement within a six to eight week period it probably won't work for you. **Cartilade** is the shark cartilage recommended by the Dr. I. William Lane researcher and author of "Sharks

Don't Get Cancer." Cartilade is either taken orally or by retention enema, or both.

An extracted protein product called "Neovastat" has shown the most promise as a topical showing an anti-inflammatory effect on lesions.

One Vitamin/Mineral Program

X-ORI™ is a program from Europe which consists of vitamins and minerals. A cream, shampoo and capsules complete a necessary regimen of internal and external assistance. X-ORI™ capsules are structured to inhibit the metabolism of arachidonic acid. People suffering from psoriasis have eight times as high a content of arachidonic acid in their skin lesions as compared with normal skin. The result, as this product claims, is that you will have more normal cell function and decline of symptoms.

16 Fasting: Clearing the Mind and Body without starving

The healthiest "supplement" to the diet of a full grown adult (25 years+) is "fasting." You can fast by abstaining from eating for a few days at a time, on a regular basis, or by not eating on a selected day every week.

Note: People with a low level of glucose in their blood, such as hypoglycemics, or with certain diseases, such as diabetes, should not attempt 100% fasts, or alter their diet without first consulting their medical caregiver.

The following excerpts are from a book by Dr. Allan Cott titled Fasting as a *Way of Life*. (He also wrote about fasting in another book titled Fasting: The Ultimate Diet).

> "I've never felt so well, I've never been so thin, I've never had so much free time."

> "I now have greater respect for my body's intelligence and capability. Fasting is a marvelous life-lesson."

> "Once I got rid of the cultural hang-up that I've got to eat all the time, fasting was a snap."

These are typical expressions reflecting the ease, comfort, and even exhilaration of the fasting experience.

Yet fasting remains controversial. There are still those whose attitudes toward going without food for even one day are frozen in fear and ignorance.

Incredibly, some doctors still believe it is "dangerous" for anyone to abstain from a single meal.

It apparently needs to be said over and over again: Fasting is not starving.

> *The body has in reserve at least a month's supply of food. It nourishes itself during a fast as if it were continuing to receive food. When this stockpile is consumed, the body signals by the return of appetite that it is time to start the refeeding program.*
>
> *Dr. George Cahill, Jr, of the Harvard School of Medicine, put the crucial fact in a nutshell: "Man's survival is predicated upon a remarkable ability, to conserve the relatively limited body protein stored, while utilizing fat as the primary-producing food."*
>
> *The body does not consume itself in any vital way even during an extended fast. This is the principal difference between the life-enhancing act of fasting and the self-destructive act of starving.*
>
> *Any so-called hunger 'pangs' are simply normal gastric contractions or stomach spasms. They represent the sensation of hunger rather than true hunger. Much of what we think of as hunger is really the desire for sensual nourishment and for pleasure and for warmth and for affection and for relief from boredom, frustration or loneliness.*
>
> *To a very large extent, "hunger" is a conditioned reflex. ('If it's noon, I must be hungry and therefore I must eat.")*
>
> *False appetite and stomach rumblings in the first few days are fleeting. They can be immediately quieted with a glass of water (You should drink a minimum of two quarts of water every day of the fast.)*
>
> *You will not feel weak or faint. In fact, you may discover new reservoirs of strength and vitality.*

I have fasted several times over many years. All the fasts were of moderate length. The longest fast was for 5-1/2 days. The first day was a little challenging. The second day was quite difficult. The third day was a little tough. The fourth and fifth were the easiest. I resumed eating according to the program I was on. You develop your fasting so you can progressively and cautiously extend the length while meeting the needs of your body and mind.

My fasting has often taken the form of drinking only fluids one day a week. I drink only water or fruit juices during this one day. When I am on a true fast I only drink water and plenty of it.

When one fasts or refrains from eating, you cause the entire digestive and elimination systems to slow down tremendously. While this slowdown can be beneficial, it also creates a problem. The existing toxins are not being removed. This causes people that are fasting to have headaches, bad breath, and general malaise. Colonic Therapy (see the chapter on: A Healthy Colon and Ways to Improved Health) during a fast produces rapid elimination of the toxins, thus enabling the fast to do what it was meant to do - rejuvenate your system.

My fasting experiences made me feel refreshed, lose a few pounds and I became more attuned to my body's needs. I truly can recommend intelligent fasting as a way of life.

Many of us have heard or read that it is healthier to be a leaner individual. Dr. Roy L. Walford, Professor of Pathology at the University of California at Los Angeles is a pioneer in caloric-restriction studies. The following information is excerpted from an article about his work.

> *Dr Walford believes we can increase the human lifespan to about 140 years or so if serious calorie-cutting starts by early adulthood. Although the benefits seem to increase with the number of calories banished (up to a point), even moderate-restriction gains extra years.*
>
> *Instead of counting calories, Dr Walford focuses on weight loss, which is safest when it takes place gradually over four to six years. He advises a target weight that's 10-25 percent below your "setpoint" the amount you weigh when you neither undereat nor overindulge. He also recommends a nutrient-packed diet reinforced with supplementary vitamins and minerals, most at officially recommended levels.*

(© Copyright reprint permission granted by Roy L. Walford, M.D.)

Another article about Dr. Walford's work, titled "Eat Less, Live Longer" by Joel N. Shurkin, appeared in the L.A. Times on March 29, 1992.

> *The way to reach this potential fountain of youth is with food - much less of it.*
>
> *While Walford waits for approval to try the regimen on humans, he is trying it out on a human guinea pig - himself. After several*

years of eating about 30% to 40% fewer calories than the average American of his height - he consumes between 1,500 and 2,000 calories a day - Walford reports he's feeling just fine. The 66-year-old scientist has lost 20 pounds during his experiment and now carries 140 pounds on his 5' 8" frame.

Walford's calorie-restriction program involves not only reducing the number of calories he consumes but also being selective about what kind of calories they are. He believes, this shrunken version of a health-food diet might not only save lives but extend them. Many scientists notice what he eats resembles the diet that's recommended for fighting heart disease.

This whole subject is a kind of taboo, Walford says. Mankind has had problems thinking about death, and has different ways of not thinking about it, like religion, philosophy. This comes over to medical professionals too. They don't want to touch anything that has to do with aging unless it's 100% proven. If you look at a general view of medicine, about 50% of (treatment) that's prescribed is not proven, it's a consensus.

Another problem impeding human experimentation is that no one knows how dietary restriction works in slowing aging. Walford thinks it prevents the natural autoimmune response of senescence, in which the body begins destroying its own tissue, and increases the ability of the DNA in the cells to repair itself. He says he has bio-chemical evidence to support that view.

(© Copyright reprint permission granted by Joel N. Shurkin)

At the time of this writing, Dr. Roy L. Walford was involved in the Biosphere 2 project. He was about halfway through a two year stint in a sealed environment (self sufficient society). The structure, in the desert, is sealed with no physical contact with the outside world. His approval came through his associate who communicated with Dr. Walford by phone and computer.

My grandmother fasted one day a month most of her life. She died at the age of 92. My mother also practiced fasting and has past her 75th birthday.

I remember an old Russian proverb, as told to me by my mother... "Have BREAKFAST with a friend, Eat LUNCH alone, Give DINNER to your enemy."

17 A Healthy Colon: Internal Washing Cleanses the Body

Colonics

Colonic irrigation is like giving a bath to the inside of your system. Irrigation flushes out poisons including pesticides, hormones and antibiotics from foods we eat, and pollution we breathe, drink and eat daily. About 26 gallons of water (during the whole session) are used with slight pressure to cleanse the length of the colon. You wash out stale bile and putrefied wastes which are poisoning your system. The average colonic visit takes about one hour and it is painless.

A colonic is a simple, easy washing of the colon, often accompanied by a light massage to the abdominal area of the body. One piece of tubing is carefully inserted in the rectum. Water flows in from a colon irrigation machine. When a client feels pressure, the therapist empties the colon into the drain. This procedure takes place many times within an hour. Everything is clean, sterilized, odorless and professionally done.

After you have completed a colonic, the therapist will give you a few capsules to replenish your colon with friendly bacteria.

According to Dr. Baum, the indigestible portion of the food you eat lodges in the large intestine and stays there until eliminated in a bowel movement. However, infrequent movements or periods of constipation can result in a partial decomposition of these waste substances which encrusts the colon and further hinders elimination. These toxins are then reabsorbed into the bloodstream, lowering the body's defenses against bacteria and viruses. The body strains to fight against the poisons, and, if the effort is too great, various organs or even the circulatory system itself can break down. The early indications of this futile war against waste, include sallow skin, nervous irritability, coated tongue, bad breath, offensive body odor, headaches, bloating, poor appetite, and a feeling of stomach heaviness.

Dr. Baum stated colonics might not be necessary if Americans had enough bulk in their diets, exercised regularly, and avoided the chemical toxins contained in alcohol, tobacco, polluted air, and processed goods. Colonics aren't designed to cure any ailment, rather they're designed to tune up the system so it becomes more capable of healing itself.

Dr. Maurice Kowan says the large bowel, or colon, is a natural sewage reservoir and is the most abused organ of the entire body. The colon has no sensory nerves to warn us, so it suffers in silence when mistreatment is heaped upon it in an effort to make it function. The colon is a highly efficient absorptive organ which, at times, floods the body with the harmful end-products of putrefactive excreta. A normal healthy colon evacuates its contents two to three times in 24 hours. One evacuation daily is not sufficient for optimum health.

Colonic therapy can remove buildup of fecal matter layers on the walls of the intestine that can collect over the years. Also, colonics clean only the colon and do not disturb any other organ or the digestive process. The treatment is relaxing, refreshing and beneficial to your health.

Enemas

Enemas are quite useful in stimulating the colon, but can be habit forming and destroy the normal reflex of the colon. However, they are a most useful and valuable tool at times. Enemas clean only the lower part of the colon and can put stress on the anal muscles.

Laxatives

People that are prone to constipation should use natural laxatives. Most fruits and vegetables aid in a healthy working digestive and elimination system. Certain foods are a little more effective, for example, apples, figs, grapes, honey, prunes, spinach, strawberries and some herbal teas. Many health food stores carry gentle and healthy laxatives. The best solution is always to improve your eating habits and learn to relax more. Sulflax is a laxative frequently recommended by Edgar Cayce.

Habits to keep you healthy include:

- Cultivate bowel movements two or three times a day
- Cultivate bowel movements at the same time each day
- A daily diet to include some form of acidophilus
- Skin brush before every shower or bath for lymph system stimulation (be sure to exclude any areas of your skin that may be irritated)
- Do squatting exercises every other day (2-3 minutes) especially during difficult bowel movement periods
- Drink at least 1 medium glass of water every 2 hours you are awake (adjust as needed)

The Welles Step

The Welles Step is a simple solution to aid individuals in bowel evacuation. The following is an explanation given in the promotional pamphlet that came with this simple and useful device:

> *People were intended to squat. They squatted throughout history. With this posture the abdominal wall and bowel are supported as we bear down. This is nature's way.*
>
> *The modern toilet was a great mistake. It leaves these two areas - the abdominal wall and bowel - unsupported as we bear down. The negative results include: incomplete elimination, a kinked bowel causing fecal stagnation, toxins entering the bloodstream, hemorrhoids and varicose veins, and a diseased colon and body.*
>
> *The Welles Step benefits include: complete bowel evacuation, freedom from laxatives, fewer hemorrhoids and hernias, fewer varicose veins, and a clean bloodstream and vibrant health.*
>
> *The device slips easily under the toilet when not in use.*

(© Copyright reprint permission granted by Welles Enterprises)

The Welles Step is a U-shaped device that can be used while sitting on most North American style toilets. The device allows you to place your feet on top of the step so your body is put into a more natural position for evacuation. I have used this inexpensive and simple device a few years and find it to be an effective aid to healthy elimination.

Internal Cleansing Program

There are a variety of cleansing programs on the market. I've used a few and find most do a good job. I have read the books and used the programs of Robert Gray, Bernard Jensen and Linda Berry and they all gave good results. Also, I found what program worked most effectively with my lifestyle - which encouraged me to maintain the program once I started.

The program I use is the "Holistic Horizon by Robert Gray" (bulking agent in powder form). Or "Perfect 7" intestinal cleanser consisting of six capsules 2 to 3 times a day, with two large glasses of water, each dose followed by 2 to 3 tablets of "Holistic Horizon by Robert Gray" intestinal cleansing formula. Also, I supplement this with a good acidophilus. I continue this program for two to three months with a few colonics strategically scheduled.

Psyllium, a grain grown mainly in India, is the main ingredient of a variety of bulking agents, intestinal cleansers and laxatives.

Elliott Douglas Derzaph

18 Mind and Body together again: Mental Exercises

Taking responsibility for your whole life is a difficult task. No matter how successful you are, there are always activities you would prefer passing to someone else in order to prevent making mistakes. Sometimes, in retrospect, you cannot believe you made such errors. I have never met anyone irrespective of age, experience, wisdom or capabilities who have accepted responsibility for their life in one easy lesson.

Maturity and respect are the truly earned areas of life. Having all the money in the world will not give you maturity or grant you the respect of others. To put it another way, success doesn't make you responsible or ensure that you can make a proper choice or make a win/win decision. Anyone who studies science, realizes that the universe is set up with an infinite number of balances, in which everything affects everything else. Whether you call it destiny, fate, karma, an action/reaction, really doesn't matter. Whenever any decision is to be made, be sure that you are making the best decision, using all you know and understand. Whatever part you did not consider or ignored could easily "bite you in the butt" and the consequences might not be pleasant.

We, in America, are fortunate in having (or had) some of the best motivators in the world - people like Norman Vincent Peale, Zig Ziglar, Anthony Robbins and Jim Rohn. These people have created their own path and planted seeds into the minds of individuals striving to see the vast possibilities in their own lives. In seeking direction with my health, I came upon many sources and have attempted to glean thoughts that may apply to our challenge.

The following are some thoughts by Louise Hay regarding a healthy new future. The information is from her best selling book - *You Can Heal Your Life*.

The Problem: Psoriasis

Probable Cause: Fear of being hurt. Deadening the senses and the self Refusing to accept responsibility for our own feelings.

New Thought Pattern: I am alive to the joys of living. I deserve and accept the very best in life. I love and approve of myself.

People vary in the value they gain from affirmations. The non-thinking or unconscious recital of words will have little value. Thinking through the *meaning* of each thought pattern on a regular basis can be valuable in each of the subject areas you wish to dominate your thinking.

NLP Comprehensive, of Boulder, Colorado, in their booklet, *A Pocket Guide to NLP - NLP: The New Technology of Achievement* stated the following:

> *Described as "software for your brain," it allows you to automatically tap into the kinds of experiences you want to have.*
>
> *You can create your own future, and you can have choices about your feelings, especially when it matters most.*

(© NLP Comprehensive. 2897 Valmont Rd., Boulder CO 80301. All Rights Reserved. Reprinted by permission.)

Dr. Kabat-Zinn of The Center for Mindfulness offers a cassette of 20 minutes designed to help psoriasis patients practice meditation and mindfulness. The centers research is geared to help people with chronic pain and stress-related disorders. Stress is a major factor in the lives of people with psoriasis. Research is still going on and participation would be appreciated. You may purchase the above cassette and the books by Dr. Kabat-Zinn.

UV treatment combined with relaxation tapes (mindfulness meditation and visualization) was 3.8 times faster than for those using light treatment alone. (Per University of Massachusetts Medical Center Study)

Our thinking can create a health hazard through stress which in turn causes flaring. Therefore, we should understand that the reverse is also true, which is relaxed, focused thinking that can improve our health.

MY AFFIRMATIONS

- I approve of myself.
- We are meant to be different.
- I am responsible for my life.
- I am willing to release the need for psoriasis.
- I release all resistance to finding a cure.
- I am grateful for what I have.

- My organs are producing the appropriate amount of fresh, clear and healthy skin.
- I have robust expectations.
- The only real success is living the life you imagine.
- I strive for progress - not perfection.
- I enjoy living a healthy relaxed life.
- I deserve and accept the very best in life.

In his booklet/catalog Valley of the Sun: *Tape Instruction and Idea Manual*, Dick Sutphen talks about achieving altered states of consciousness through the use of hypnosis, meditation and relaxation:

> *Sometimes the explanations aren't even logical.*
> *For example, the case study of Nancy, who had a terrible case of atopic dermatitis, a chronic skin condition that leaves your skin with itchy open sores. Practically everything aggravated her condition: too much sun, too much sweat, too much soap. Nancy had borne the disease since childhood, and doctors told her she could expect to bear it for the rest of her life.*
> *As a last resort, she went into an altered state of consciousness and asked herself the question, "Why am I creating this skin condition for myself?" The answer she received was: "One of the primary lessons you want to learn in this life is to be sensitive and open to other people. You choose to have a super-sensitive exterior - your skin - to remind you to reveal your even more sensitive interior - your true Self. When you do this, your skin condition will disappear."*
> *After coming back to full consciousness, Nancy stated that, although logically she shouldn't believe a word of it, for some reason it felt right. She admitted that she never allowed her true Self to be exposed to others for fear of rejection.*
> *Several months later Nancy wrote to say that, since that session, she had followed her own advice and began revealing herself to others who became her friends. Her skin condition had cleared up entirely.*

(© Copyright reprint permission granted by Valley of the Sun, Malibu, CA)

It has been said repeatedly that your **knowledge, education and experience** contribute 15% toward accomplishing your goal, and **attitude** accounts for the other 85%. **What you do**, with what you know, determines your degree of success. Your choices define a direction that works specifically to develop your view of the world. The appreciation you have of life determines the extent to which your goals will be fulfilled.

Each of us has our Jacob's ladder or cross to bear. I choose to think of life's offerings, that affect us personally in terms of challenges. Mario Cuomo, a governor of the state of New York, may have said it best, "The game is lost only when we stop trying."

I wish you good fortune with all your goals.

Elliott Douglas Derzaph

19 Healing Imagery: Seeing Yourself Clearly

A simple tool, used very little in our society, is "imagery." Imagery is the mind thinking in pictures. You would use imagery to produce in your mind a set of clear, conscious pictures of the health goal you want to achieve.

I am sure many have heard the metaphor that life is like a movie. The only problem is that most of us do not realize that we are the producer, the director and the actors running the entire show. By allowing ourselves to become habituated in our thinking, we walk away from our own "movie" forgetting that the "movie (our life)" never stops.

In our mind, we can do anything we want. Our mind is what produces all we have in this world, including our bodies. We need to produce a series of pictures in our mind that clearly show the healthy state we want both inside and outside our body.

You may have read that people like Norman Cousins pioneered public knowledge of the benefits of imagery. He is a living testament to its success. As a doctor and patient at UCLA he used imagery to cure himself of the deadly disease of cancer; and thus led the way for many others to help themselves with a variety of diseases, using the same techniques.

Imagery has been used successfully throughout the ages to produce a whole spectrum of benefits, from the material (such as acquiring wealth) to the mental (such as repairing physical, psychological or emotional problems). Your ability to pay full attention and concentrate singlemindedly while being in a relaxed and stress free state is necessary to achieve the desired results.

In the marketplace, you will find instruction from many sources describing the use of imagery to achieve a multitude of goals. Sometimes when you observe the workings of an event you will see imagery being used, yet the presenters and/or participants will not be aware, or at least will not bring out the fact, that imagery is being practiced.

NLP holds that people think and act based on their internal representations of the world and not on the world itself. Once we understand specifically how we create and maintain our inner thoughts and feelings, it is a simple matter for us to change them to more useful ones.

A clear sequence of mental pictures of what you want and the repetition of these pictures will produce favorable results. Keep in mind that the problem did not develop overnight and the solution will not be achieved overnight. Be patient, consistent and always be progressive in your thinking. Work toward small goals to ensure that you achieve a modicum of success before attempting to solve your biggest challenges in life.

Imagery is very useful in dealing with all kinds of difficulties we have as humans. Imagery uses your unconscious memory ability to frame a visual thought which can constantly and instantly guide your conscious thoughts towards a chosen path.

What follows is a quick overview of imagery:

a. Remember clearly a familiar memory which is out of order with the accomplishment of a goal. (Example: an error, etc.)

b. Create in your mind a crystal clear picture of what you want to **replace** that erroneous thought.

c. Create a sequence of pictures in your mind starting with where you **are,** and ending with where you **want to be.**

d. Daily - **see** these pictures clearly in your mind until they unfold into life.

Be sure of what you want because you will get exactly what you think about.

No imagery details should be eliminated and all aspects should be clearly understood to obtain the impact and consequences it is capable of achieving.

Interactive Guided Imagery is a refined version of imagery. Using the mind-body premise and the view that the unconscious contains all the details necessary to solve disorders such as illnesses. You need to take the information in your unconscious and move it to your conscious mind. This process can be done by yourself but it is difficult. It is recommended that you use a therapist initially to get the most out of this natural therapy. The Academy for Guided Imagery can be contacted for practitioners, books and tapes. The Academy is located in Mill Valley, California and can be reached at 800-726-2070 or 415-389-9324.

Hypnosis

A 1997 Johns Hopkins study found that *some* patients who underwent hypnosis (including skeptics) visualized their condition clearing up on its own and enjoy a complete remission of symptoms, even among those that were skeptics. Therefore, hypnosis may be ideal for some psoriasis sufferers. For referrals, send a (self addressed stamped envelope) to the American Society of Clinical Hypnosis, 130 East Elm Court, Suite 201, Roselle, IL 60172-2000; 630-980-4740 or email: info@asch.net.

20 Freeing Dis-Ease: The Path To Emotional Intelligence®

I begin this section of the book by explaining an important understanding that my own 25+ years of experience with psoriasis has provided.

First, emotions are, and always will be, a major factor in our health. Second, our personal observations (perhaps assessed by others with insight in our lives) are necessary to turn the tide of any disease or challenge we encounter in life. And third, very important in such observation is the identification of the personal "triggers" that transform ordinary difficulties into emotional crises that stress our organs and our bodies to the point that a loss of health results.

Thus, I found that my personal trigger - the situation that produces overpowering stress in my mind - is "financial distress." When I encounter financial distress at a level that makes me feel overwhelmed, I will have a psoriasis outbreak, irrespective of the measures I may be taking to maintain good health or be psoriasis free. This sequence - stress as a result of financial difficulties, followed by a psoriasis outbreak - is as predictable as the ticking of a Swiss watch. With this knowledge in hand, I am confident I will be able to find the tools to resolve a lifetime of reactions to this "trigger." Other psoriasis sufferers must be able to find their "trigger" and be aptly prepared to deal with it to reduce the severity of the disease.

A wise old friend named Thane told me something many years ago, *"There are two things an individual needs before he can expect to be of value to him/herself or anyone or anything else in this world. They must first and foremost be sane. And then they must be healthy. If a person cannot help themselves and have the qualities of a sane individual then he can't possibly be of help to others."*

Ray Jobling is National Chairman of the Psoriasis Association of Great Britain wrote in an article titled "Psoriasis keeps you thinking." He wrote, on the famous authors John Updike and Dennis Potter who both had Psoriasis. Ray wrote "As so movingly revealed in the literary works of Updike and Potter, major skin disorders can be deeply stigmatizing. Living with such conditions is as much a matter of emotions, feelings and relationships as it is of reasoned understanding and calculated physical therapy." Also, Ray wrote "Those with chronic skin conditions have to be more self-aware." The American writer, John Updike who had Psoriasis since early childhood. He says, "The name of the disease, spiritually speaking, is humiliation." Jerry Mathers of "Leave it to Beaver" fame has Psoriasis and is a spokesman for the public education of Psoriasis.

After many years of intensive research into the body-mind connection, Bill Moyers completed a book, and a PBS series entitled "Healing and the Mind." Moyers' research included interviews with medical experts, in fields ranging from neurology and immunology to acupuncture and massage. Moyers investigated how thoughts and feelings influence health and how healing relates to the mind. He concluded: *"There are many, many reasons to believe that the connection is strong and that this link has a profound effect on our physical, emotional and spiritual well-being."*

There are a variety of factors that contribute to your health... and to your psoriasis. Most health experts agree that your emotions play a significant part in your well being. The greatest professional help in the world will not aid anyone unwilling to help themselves in a sane fashion. This chapter concerns itself primarily with your emotional health. The bottom line is that *you* control your well being.

Most psoriasis patients have a greater challenge dealing with the appearance of psoriasis than with the continual treatment, though, that too can be monotonous and frustrating at times.

First, it is very important to be honest and open with yourself about psoriasis. Then, you must be open with family and friends. The first step in dealing with any challenge in life is facing the realities and obtaining the support needed to achieve a workable solution. Touching, physically and verbally, is an important step.

I used to tell people all kinds of things when someone referring to my psoriasis would ask, "What is that?" If a person appeared pleasant, I might say it was just a rash. However, if I felt any discomfort with their question, I might say it was skin cancer or AIDS or leprosy. In the past I had always felt better keeping people at arms length, both figuratively and literally.

It's important to feel and express how psoriasis influences you. It is perfectly O.K. to think and feel and say what is going on within you. Getting your emotions out in a sane fashion will not only help you, but will help everyone with whom you come into contact. Find someone - a friend, a member of your family, or a professional counselor - to listen to you. Find someone who will let you hear what you are saying and allow you to resolve it within yourself. Then, you need to accept, and diligently follow, your own path of workable solutions. To be aware of a difficulty and realize you must do something about it is a hugely successful beginning. Your commitment to the important values in your life will allow you to be your best.

You must accept the reality of psoriasis. You must be the one in control. If you aren't, then the psoriasis governs your life. It is always your choice which runs the show.

Successfully confronting your psoriasis can open the door to other emotionally charged areas in your life. This *step-exposing other emotionally charged areas* - can be an opportunity to overcome other difficulties of importance. These problems can also be sanely challenged and resolved to the best of your ability, either by yourself or, when needed, with the help of professionals.

Find a dermatologist who shows genuine interest and concern for you. He/she should be open to new ideas in the marketplace or from you. A physician who cares will be beneficial to you now and in the future. Be responsible for your treatment using the physician as a professional guide.

The main responsibility of the dermatologist is to get your skin as clear as possible, with the best methods available, under the safest possible conditions.

No sane person intends to hurt himself/herself or others as a result of his/her difficulties in life. But I have found one emotional challenge to which we, as Americans, fall victim. Those in the business world, in the world of sports and many others, including those with a disease have many times given the unfortunate impression, that if you are not outstanding in your class, that you count for very little. I believe this attitude to be, in itself, a diseased emotional state. Everyone, who tries to the best of their ability, deserves full credit. I am sure whatever created us didn't intend for us to lock ourselves away when problems arose or when we came in second or third, instead of first.

We were given a life for only one purpose ... to live it to the best of our ability. That means learning to love our fellow-man enough to forgive his errors or ignorance and to allow ourselves the very same right to be loved and forgiven.

At the completion of the first draft of this book, I fractured my right leg. This required that I use crutches and wear a cast for two months. When I removed the cast I found the bottom of my foot covered with a layer of thick, cracked skin. I thought it was dead skin - like a callus. During my recovery using just an aircast, I had no thought 'this could be psoriasis'. Within three weeks my foot was back to a normal healthy appearance. Then, when I was editing this book, I found some photographs of psoriasis of the feet. It looked exactly like my foot did upon removing the cast. I am certain my attitude of "this is dead skin and not psoriasis" affected the healing process.

Elliott Douglas Derzaph

Many believe stress is the cause for up to fifty percent of psoriasis outbreaks. Stress creates toxins within our body. A negative state of mind of any kind creates stress through a chemical change in the bloodstream. **Stress can cause an outbreak of psoriasis and psoriasis itself can cause stress. You can break this cycle.**

The following observations about stress are excerpted from Love Your Disease, a book by John Harrison, M.D.

> *The child, forced by parental pressure to make a decision he is ill equipped to make, responds with stress and makes an adaptation. Stress is a consequence of the grown-up failing to relieve his own internal little kid from the burden of the early decision.*
>
> *All illness is a consequence of stress; not stress arising from an individual's immediate environment but left over from a time in childhood when survival made an adaptation necessary.*
>
> *Stress, like illness, is assumed to be beyond the control of the individual. In reality it is self-created, and a synonym for fear.*
>
> *Stress is old fear.*

(Excerpted from Love Your Disease Copyright © 1984 by John Harrison, M.D., Hay House, Carson, Ca. Reprinted by permission.)

While having discussions with friends and relatives, I found a common denominator in their conclusions as to when and why their psoriasis first appeared and the cause of flare-ups. Their insightful conclusion was that emotional problems were the cause of psoriasis. The first place winner was some form of stress, caused by being part of a dysfunctional family, or by abuse or by financial difficulties.

When I was younger and living in Canada someone close to me made some mistakes and had the unfortunate experience of going to jail as a result. During incarceration the psoriasis completely cleared. The psoriasis did not return until rejoining society.

Reports surface regularly from the psychological world about psoriasis patients having flare-ups whenever they had emotional problems. NPF states, *"It has been observed that a change in environment will sometimes be followed by a spontaneous clearance of the psoriasis."*

Uncontrolled psoriasis in children can interfere with learning and play, and cause severe depression, anxiety and embarrassment. Always check with your doctor to ensure that the medication being used is the right strength for your children. Ensure that as soon as their health improves that you contact their health professional to get approval to discontinue the use of their medication. Sit down regularly with your children to discuss their feelings especially as it relates to psoriasis. Extra care should be taken to ensure that your child has a good attitude towards life. This good attitude can be refined with opportunities to express all emotions felt within a safe environment.

Laughter

The benefits of laughter have even been qualified by the A.M.A. as an aid to good health. Laughter has an overall benefit to the health of the body. Laughter relaxes you, pumps oxygen into your blood, stabilizes blood pressure and encourages circulation. Enjoy laughter often. It can improve your life in so many ways.

Laughter, according to Dr. Norman Cousins and many others, is the key to good health. Also, it can be a major healing factor for a disease. Laughter creates endorphins, a product created to aid the body in recovering from disease.

Anger and Challenging Emotions

Anger seems the most common emotional expression in psoriasis patients. Learning to sanely face and express this anger can be a turning point in dealing with psoriasis. In the following pages, I offer a variety of methods to help you deal with psoriasis emotionally.

Many people and ideas in my life have directed me to a healthier and saner path. Learning to sanely and effectively release my emotions produced the most profound effect on my life.

There are many roads to the understanding and use of emotional release. Some you'll find to be quite simple, and others very complex. I will give an overview of a few just to start you off in the right direction. The intent, its intensity and self-honesty, is what creates the benefit when using these methods. The tools used to begin the process of developing your emotional side are listed below.

'Fantastic potential' is the only way to describe our emotional ability, though it is an area needing substantial work to get us from our present early stage of development and to refine a sensible process for growth. The name, I think best expresses this realm of greatness in man, is "Emotional Intelligence®." It has been said often, and I agree, "You will never encounter anything in your life that you cannot handle if you don't give up and utilize the best resources to meet your challenge."

Before starting you down the path of emotional regeneration, I will list four points made in the book, The Emotional Hostage, by Leslie Cameron-Bandler and Michael Lebeau. The points concern the problems that result if you do not express your emotions.

1. What is going on inside you fails to be conveyed to those around you. You have a message, but it stays locked inside until it erupts.

2. Allowing emotions to go unexpressed robs you of an opportunity to get what you want from those around you.

3. Not expressing your emotions is bad for your health. Personnel and medical records are filled with such examples.

4. People can't know who you are if they have no idea what you are feeling.

Sane Emotional Releases

First, the simplest and most common action, is to realize we all make mistakes and to forgive ourselves and everyone else. This is the method offered by many religions and the least effective for most of us.

Next, I present a quotation excerpted from the book *You Can Heal Your Life* by Louise L. Hay:

> *To Release the Past, We Must be Willing to Forgive.*
>
> *We need to choose to release the past and forgive everyone, ourselves included. We may not know how to forgive, and we may not want to forgive; but the very fact we say we are willing to forgive begins the healing process. It is imperative for our own healing that "we" release the past and forgive everyone.*
>
> *"I forgive you for not being the way I wanted you to be. I forgive you and I set you free."*
>
> *This affirmation sets us free.*

(Excerpted from You Can Heal Your Life. © 1984 by Louise L. Hay, Hay House, Carson, Ca. Reprinted by Permission)

Another affirmation by Ms. Hay that is useful is *"I release that which I no longer need."* Once something is no longer of value or suitable or appropriate in your life or the circumstance in which you find yourself, it is time to free oneself of that habit, activity or thinking.

N.L.P. Comprehensive offers a tape cassette program called "The Forgiveness Pattern." This series gives a brief, yet insightful, look into the realm of forgiveness. It gave me helpful ideas on how to work with my emotions and the emotions of those around me. Learning to forgive is truly the primary step in the road all of us travel to move beyond our present turmoil.

The N.L.P. tape stated forgiveness as; creating a healing connection; acquiring a commonality with others; reacquiring a connection. Forgiveness is not for that other person or the world but for you. You learn to self-forgive; then you learn to forgive others.

All people have good intentions for others and themselves. People's shortcomings are what causes erring. People do not intentionally hurt others, they just lack proper education in a specific area of their life. When a need has not been filled wisely in our lives we choose whatever resource is available to fill it though it may not always be a sane or intelligent solution.

David Harp wrote a book, *The Three Minute Meditator*, with a chapter titled "The Forgiveness Meditation," which I will now quote.

> *This one is very simple, although not always easy. Just picture someone whom you think has hurt or wronged you in some way. It's important, for now, to choose someone with whom you're no longer very angry. Visualize them as clearly as you can. And tell them, "I forgive you. I forgive you for hurting or wronging me."*
>
> *Repeat it a number of times, and try to feel forgiving, try to feel yourself giving up remnants of anger or righteousness towards them. If you are not sure with whom you're ready to do this exercise, do it with someone whose hurt to you was very minor - a driver who slipped ahead of you on the freeway, or a clerk who overcharged you by a few cents. Eventually, with practice, you'll be able to do this exercise with people who have caused you more serious pain.*
>
> *It is crucial to remember that forgiving a person does not mean that you condone or accept their behavior. You are forgiving the person, not his/her behavior. And letting go of anger, and of feelings of having been wronged, is a very freeing experience. For me, doing this exercise on the publisher who had "appropriated" my harmonica book and title concept allowed me to stop wasting energy on anger and self-hatred, and to get on with my life.*

Here is a point made by David Harp that I thought appropriate in this vein.

> Relate to another person with the understanding that the other has as many feelings and needs, fears and desires, as you do. And as much right to pursue them, instead of acting as though the other person is mostly an object, whose principal purpose in life is to help you gain satisfaction.

Meditation has been accepted in corporate America as an effective way to aid executives in dealing with stress. The practice of sitting quietly and observing yourself breathe in and out, for fifteen minutes a day, can reduce stress considerably and, for some, completely. Try it.

After many years of reading and listening, I have developed a personal philosophy with the following ideas I have found along the way:

- Practice forgiving yourself immediately for any perceived failure.

- Celebrate successes, analyze failures, and never punish yourself.

- Think, "I learned a valuable lesson and next time I'll try it like this...."

- Teach yourself to be as encouraging and imaginative in your support of your own efforts.

One of the things we should know is that even if we didn't get psoriasis we would have a 99% chance of getting another disease. Psoriasis was the manifestation caused by a disorder in our system. Look at psoriasis as something created because we pushed something in our system to the brink. The dis-ease expressed was probably selected from a DNA weak link inherited to us from our parents. (This is not to blame anyone since we all have our shortcomings).

THE NEXT STEP TO WELLNESS

The school of thought which is gaining increasing credibility are ontologically based which states there are psychological and emotional components not only underlying illness but the conditions and circumstances of one's life. You can track the persistent evolution of this new movement toward wellness in the ever-widening acceptance and utilization of alternative methods of healing and self-fulfillment.

I consider myself to be extremely fortunate that my own personal exploration of such alternative methodologies like the study of Ontology (scientific philosophical thinking) led me to a school of thought that has been on the cutting edge of such breakthroughs which is to me the single most advanced and sophisticated approach to the transformation of the human condition in the world today.

The school's approach to the important arena of self-transformation and personal development was to integrate the highest and best of Eastern and Western traditions while discarding superfluous and unsafe practices. It is this synthesis of complementary disciplines that has resulted in the most powerfully therapeutic teaching.

This school is unique among self-improvement schools in providing a profound philosophical model of human development that is unbiased, unified, holistic and experiential. This exploration into the nature of self and reality is designed to liberate potentials latent within everyone. It is a movement toward authenticity in identity, purpose and living that can transform and uplift where you now find yourself.

This new system of self-development goes beyond the conventional mind/body hypothesis to a nondual model where no condition or situation is considered irreversible. Genuine transformation of self is requisite to the restoration of wellness in every area of life.

Note: Emotional Intelligence® is a registered trademark by the author Elliott Derzaph. Emotional Intelligence® can be described as sanely accessing an evolving kaleidoscope of infinitely diverse and boundless interacting emotions. The author has been doing research into this subject since 1974 when he met Dr. Kenneth (Thane) Walker. Anyone interested in this subject should send a letter to: Emotional Intelligence, P.O. Box 643038, Los Angeles, CA 90064-3038.

Elliott Douglas Derzaph

21 A Personal Journey

I believe personal experience is the best teacher. The depth to which you understand another person's situation depends on how personally and emotionally you become involved in their experience. In this chapter, I will share moments in my history that may have value beyond the physical nuts and bolts of psoriasis.

During my story, I will pay attention to the major negative incidents of my life. Since I understand that positive emotional incidents create a healthy change or effect in the body, we are looking for those incidents that may have somehow caused the body to fail along the way.

We will keep in mind that psoriasis is hereditary and ask the question, "What is it that causes one person in a family to get psoriasis while your brother or sister doesn't?" Is it emotions? I think emotions are a major key to who develops psoriasis. You will find many doctors and patients referring to psoriasis as "red, inflamed and angry."

I am an American citizen, though I was born in 1953 in a small city in Canada, just a few miles north of the American border. My parents both worked hard developing the family business.

Unfortunately, my father was to find out, too late, that his partner had embezzled all the company's funds. He was also to find out that some family members had been cheating the company for years. Shortly after his discoveries the business collapsed. My father took up drinking and socially acceptable abusive behavior. I love my father, but, he had been challenged by alcoholism for more than thirty years.

Unfortunately, drinking and hitting members of your family was quite common in those days and tolerated by most of the public. Many people talked of the pain it caused but never seemed to find any acceptable solutions. It all appeared to be the way life was lived. Many people just put up with it. I now know it was fortunate my parents parted when they did.

My parents separated when I was seventeen. My father went into a rehabilitation center for help. The program wasn't as successful as hoped. My mother had my two younger brothers to care for and little money with which to do it. She also wanted to get as far away as possible. She asked if I wanted to go with her but I knew she really couldn't afford it. I felt everyone was abandoning my father even though I knew he was abusive.

Until that time I was known as a "nice young man," and I was very active in sports. But, after I went out on my own, I took up smoking, drinking to excess, and drugs.

Also, I started dating frequently. Then, I began to date someone different every night. For years, my only satisfaction was to be numb with drugs or alcohol. Sex made me feel good for only a few moments and I didn't enjoy being touched, except the minimum amount required to have sex. I would do anything to keep from being conscious of my feelings.

When I turned twenty-one, I moved to the United States. I entered college and got a job working for the Dean of Students. The Dean was also a psychoanalyst and writer; and with his help I turned my self-destructive life around. I gave up my drug and drinking habits and began living a constructive life.

I worked with the Dean for five years and then parted ways, a very difficult decision. Simultaneously, I broke off a one year relationship with my girlfriend who had a drinking problem and with whom I had great difficulty living. I moved again, this time to Northern California. I spent eight months helping a retired businesswoman remodel her newly acquired house on the Bay. During that time, I enjoyed a non-sexual but very satisfying relationship with another woman, who had been dealt an unfair burden by her ex-boyfriend's escapades.

I couldn't see a future where I was, so I moved in with some friends living on the west side of Los Angeles. I made the move thinking the situation would be temporary. But after sleeping on the couch and looking for a job for months and not being able to make any new friends, I got quite discouraged.

Again, I took up drinking and non-commitment relationships. It appeared I was coming up empty-handed in all I undertook. My discouragement got the best of me and I stupidly consumed large quantities of drugs and alcohol. I lost such control that I found myself, disoriented, in the care of a friend. I had been asleep for several days due to the combined effect of the alcohol and drugs. With the help of friends and professional counseling, I turned my life around. I never again saw any value in giving up.

During all this time I had become quite a success with women... and developed an ego of comparable size. I could convince a woman to give me her phone number and go on a date, all within two minutes of meeting her for the first time. Yet, I couldn't understand why I wasn't able to make the relationships last more than two or three months.

Now, twenty five years old, I found that I had developed plaque psoriasis. For years the psoriasis was very minor and did not have any noticeable effect on my life-style or on those with whom I interacted.

At the age of thirty three, my psoriasis started to spread more rapidly. I was living with a woman who accepted me, with my psoriasis. We had worked out many of our difficulties, but had not resolved her drinking problem. Finally, I realized that I maintained the turbulent relationship because of caring for the children and soon thereafter I ended the relationship.

About this same time, I came to realize that a few women were judging me by my psoriasis. For years, I had been judging women by their bodies and now the tables had been turned and I was being judged by the way my body looked. This included a nurse who told me she couldn't date me again because of my psoriasis. I have to admit I was quite shocked upon hearing that.

About a year later, I finally realized that a long term relationship - though not necessarily marriage - was what I wanted in my life. Slowly, my relationships started improving. I realized that friendship needed to precede the establishment of any long-term relationship. After a few more bumps, I came to believe that a marriage based on friendship, communication and a few solid goals could be very satisfying and successful.

Within a couple of weeks of my new realizations; and after conversing with many of the females in my "little black book," I decided to eliminate from consideration all the women I already knew. Shortly after clearing my phone book, I made new friends. I promised myself that I wouldn't go on even one date without first being able to have intelligent discussions of mutual interest over the telephone. Although not my intention, these discussions continued - without dating - for many months. I discovered I had no patience for anyone who was not ready to make a full-time commitment to a new relationship.

I conversed with Wendy, a new friend, for months before our first date although this long delay was not intentional. Our careers kept at least one of us constantly out of town or busy with other commitments. We met for the first time six months after our first contact. I must admit it turned out amazingly well. I fell in love immediately. Wendy has the most beautiful heart and mind of any friend I have ever met.

From our first date, we knew we wanted to be with each other and from that point on we were always together. I proposed marriage to Wendy, exactly one year after our first date. We married one year and three weeks after that. Wendy accepted whatever came with me. This includes her experiencing my psoriasis worsening as the wedding date approached. My psoriasis was at its worst in my whole life, just days before our wedding.

I discovered only recently that for many years I was unconsciously using my psoriasis as a convenient, but foolish method of harnessing my ego. My studies and interests required that I look more closely at myself and answer the question: Why do you do the things you do? I realized I was my own biggest problem and how I was standing in my own way. I am the only one who knows exactly the solution to the unique and complex mix of problems I have created in my world. I have to solve my own problems, at my own pace, to make the world better for myself.

I strongly believe that I used my psoriasis to teach myself a little humility. And I used it to test the caring or love of women I met. I felt that if they could accept my psoriasis they could surely accept the rest of me. And finally came the biggest test of all. "Would someone marry me while my psoriasis was very noticeable and at its worst in my life?" The answer was, "yes!.."

I have found a loving family and true friends. Also, I have come to discover that any reasonably humane person will be accepting and caring even though you may have psoriasis. I think psoriasis has been a significant character building experience in my life.

I am sharing my history only because, I believe emotions play a major part in your being healthy or having "dis-eases" of mind and body; and, I wanted you, the reader, to see how much of a part my emotions played in the development of my disease.

I have had psoriasis for more than twenty-four years. This includes the thirteen+ years I have known my wife. Upon completion of this book and submitting it to my publisher a wonderful thing happened. My psoriasis cleared up. For the first time in all the years I have known my wife, she can now see my soma in a way I had only dreamt of. She can touch my skin without my thinking of how my psoriasis looks or feels, because it is finally gone. I know not if, or when, or how intense the psoriasis will be in my life again.

I don't know for sure, whether the writing of this book alone reduced my stress level, which in turn, slowed down my outbreaks and then relieved me of any psoriatic plaques! But I do know it wasn't a coincidence.

The family members who have given their help, love and support for those with Psoriasis I would like to express the greatest of thanks and wish all of you the best of health.

Elliott Douglas Derzaph

22 Conclusions: Evolution of Our Hopes

Time does not stand still. Technology and science is always changing and developing; and the facts of yesterday do not consistently hold true today. Who can determine what tomorrow holds for us? As an example, prior to 1995, researchers' view of psoriasis was that it was a skin cell disorder. In 1995, that view was changed and psoriasis was considered to be an immunologic disorder. Currently, NPF has encouraged clinical research toward the emerging model, which points to psoriasis as an autoimmune disorder. Thus, what we have found to be helpful today could be totally obsolete within a year. It appears that we must be flexible and open-minded in our pursuit of the resolution of any illness we might have today. What might work for us today may not work next week but, more importantly, is the fact that tomorrow definitely has a solution which will make psoriasis a thing of the past. It is encouraging to know that over 30 companies have drugs in testing to treat Psoriasis.

I found psoriasis patients have common denominators, though there will be inconsistency in terms of a single, well defined cause. Psoriasis treatment demands different treatments for different individuals. Or back to, "What works for some may not work for others." Find what works for you; and if or when necessary, alter your choice. It is important to remember that optimum health is usually acquired with an overall plan and trusting and believing your efforts definitely make a difference. Remember, psoriasis is not contagious or deadly and, for the most part, is controllable.

A blend of sunlight, moisture, lack of stress, a method for sane emotional release, activity that stretches the body while keeping the spine flexible, and eating habits which develop a body that is lean and healthy... this combination, I believe, will create the environment to aid the resolution of psoriasis on an individual basis. If an overall view is one of building and maintaining our physical and mental health, we will place ourselves in the optimum position for achieving a solution to our psoriasis!

One choice which clearly appears to be significant in dealing effectively with psoriasis is our emotions. We have found negative emotions wreak havoc in the body, resulting in disease. Keep in mind that emotions govern our thought processes; and consider the effect that has on our psychological makeup - who we think we are. If the negative emotions are not dealt with, the disease will return and continue to deteriorate the body and mind.

Psoriasis: The Struggle and the Triumph
A Healthy Transformation for Everyone Living with Psoriasis

On the other side, positive emotions build the strength needed for a healthy body. Learning emotional control or emotional appropriateness or simply having emotionally sane intercourse is the savior of our health. "Emotional Intelligence®" is obscure to more than 99.99% of the world's population. Taking advantage of every opportunity to use sane, emotional expression will not only aid the individual but all of society. Take time regularly to share your thoughts and feelings with a friend.

You are the only person who can make yourself healthy. You must be the one who takes control of your health. The interactions among yourself, your doctors and the rest of your world can provide the blend of intelligent and caring direction to fully satisfy your health needs. Only one person cares enough about you, to do the very best for you... YOU.

The following two paragraphs are excerpted from the epilogue of the book, Love Your Disease, by John Harrison, M.D.:

> *To cure ourselves we need to take back the responsibility of loving and caring for ourselves from whomever we have entrusted the task. We need to accept ourselves whoever, whenever and however we are. That means accepting that we have made ourselves unwell and we will care for ourselves the best way we know how. When we have taken back full responsibility for ourselves, we can then find others who will be willing to help us. We can play while we share the joys and burdens of responsibility.*
>
> *We can make use of those healing professionals, orthodox or alternative, who make themselves available. We can pass through the transition stage of partial responsibility while under the umbrella of their care. When we are ready we can risk leaving the nest and taking off on our own, knowing that we can return if we want, it is not for me, with my own needs, to tell you how, when or where you do it.*

(*Love Your Disease.* © 1984 by John Harrison, M.D. Hay House, Carson, Ca. Reprinted by permission.)

We have three fronts to manage. First, the genetic factor. Psoriasis is a genetic DNA error resulting in a predisposition to manufacture excess skin within a particular environment.

Second, the social pitfalls. The ignorance of the public and its attitude towards people with psoriasis. Reactions range from rejection to derogatory comments. The judgement of others, and then self-judgement, causes stress. (People with disabilities have greater acceptance in our society than people with psoriasis). We must deal with a social stereotype: *physical appearance matters more than the rest of you.* An individual may be emotionally, and intellectually healthy, but still be shunned by the public because of the appearance of his/her psoriasis.

And third, our eating habits. The ingredients, (food and water) for rebuilding our bodies are given minor attention by most, due to bad eating habits perpetuated by the marketplace. I suggest reading everything you can get your hands on, especially the book by the British author Dr. Caroline Wilson (to cover the basics most doctors use to work with psoriasis) and the American author Dr. John Pagano (to take a look at new ideas in working with psoriasis). I think a membership in both the National Psoriasis Foundation (U.S.) and the Canadian Psoriasis Foundation will give you the greatest access to information. It's time the healing of the body and mind were considered together, as a whole.

My intention is not to give you one specific solution, but a list of available options and areas of knowledge... a handbook for psoriasis, a book offering a system, so you will experience only minimal displeasure, discomfort and detriment from your psoriasis.

I wish each and every one of you the best life has to offer. Take care.

Psoriasis: The Struggle and the Triumph
A Healthy Transformation for Everyone Living with Psoriasis

Chapters Digest

Introductory Chapter

1. You should not put yourself totally in the hands of your doctor; you must independently obtain information about your condition, evaluate it and use it to complement suggested medical treatment. Serious problems can result if you, as a psoriasis sufferer, take no responsibility for your own treatment.

2. The National Psoriasis Foundation's "Bill of Rights" for psoriasis sufferers is reprinted with permission with a few more encompassing additions.

3. Then Dincin Buchman in her book, "Herbal Medicine," suggests altering our attitudes to include a more holistic view of diet and exercise; the detective in us should be unearthing the causes of the symptoms.

Chapter 1

1. Psoriasis affects some 8 million Americans and Canadians and 60-80 million people around the world. Onset can occur from birth throughout life; average age at onset is 27. Psoriasis is thought by some to be a disease of the autoimmune system. It is not contagious. It is reversible and relatively harmless. It can be brought under temporary control with some medical treatments. Its biggest discomforts are its appearance and a continual itching. Psoriasis is hereditary but may skip a generation. Stress is a major factor in the onset or relapse of psoriasis.

2. Treatment for psoriasis is difficult because what works once may not work again; and what works for one, may not work for another. The only treatments which work for most are general health measures including good eating habits, good emotional health, high self-concept and effective stress management.

3. The Edgar Cayce Foundation reports that the gastrointestinal tract's failings cause seepage of toxic substances into the circulatory system. The body, unable to eliminate the toxic products through the emunctory

systems, gets assistance from the lymph flow which becomes congested creating the inflammatory reaction characteristic of psoriasis.

4. Information published in 1987 describes some doctors' beliefs that psoriasis is linked to a disruption in normal cell maturation and growth. This occurs because the skin of psoriasis patients does not recognize a hormone produced by the kidney which stops the proliferation of skin cells.

Chapter 2

1. Careful removal or softening of psoriatic scales is important in speeding the beneficial effects of topically applied products.

2. Dr. Isadore Rosenfeld comments on Sulfasalazine and Sandostatin in his book "The Best Treatment." Sulfasalazine has been approved for treatment. The status of Sandostatin research is unknown.

3. Dr. Lawrence Miller comments on Zostrix in the book, Doctors Book of Home Remedies. Zostrix, made from the active ingredient in red pepper, exhausts all the body's supplies of substance P, a chemical believed to cause inflammation and which is also found in psoriatic placques.

4. Dr. Linda Berry recommends skin brushing in her book internal Cleansing - A Practical Guide to Colon Health, as the best way to cleanse the skin and lymphatic system.

5. Dr. Friedman suggests the use of watertight dressings to lock in moisture and topicals to the skin.

6. Hobe Laboratories offers "Psoria-Gard" natural ingredient skin treatment.

7. Sprays are medium in cost with a range of patient improvement at 50% to 90%.

Chapter 3

1. Sunlight is the least expensive, healthiest, rejuvenating natural product which can aid in relieving psoriasis. UVA and UVB are ultraviolet components of sunlight. Treatments are also given with artificial UVA

and UVB. Treatment with UVA usually includes the internal drug, psoralen, and is known as PUVA. Treatment with UVB usually includes topical use of tar. PUVA and ultraviolet B radiation cause damage to membranes as well as to DNA. PUVA can also alter immune responses.

2. Dead Sea sun and seawater treatments have been successful in clearing psoriasis in up to 80% of patients.

3. Home phototherapy systems are now more available and improved. You must be sure to get a doctor's approval and guidance in using these systems independently.

4. Companies which sell sunlamp equipment for home use are listed.

Chapter 4

1. Water benefits you internally by replenishing the fluids the body needs; and externally, by refreshing and supplying moisture to the skin.

2. Most soaps dry the skin at the same time they clean the skin; so soap should be completely washed off the skin before drying.

Chapter 5

1. A massage is a pleasurable experience which relaxes and invigorates us. Massages offer an array of cosmetic, physiological, and psychological benefits to the skin, the internal organs, and the body, as a whole.

2. There are many types of massage, including French, Swedish, lymphatic and polarity. Lymphatic massage stimulates the secretion of toxic wastes. Polarity massage helps put the body's energy field in balance.

Chapter 6

1. Non-invasive care is recommended when choices are available. Surgery is a last resort that should be carefully researched before proceeding. At least one or two other medical opinions should be obtained.

2. Dr. Robert Skinner comments on the use of a laser to remove patches without scarring or damaging surrounding healthy tissue. Laser treatment clears lesions permanently, in nearly all cases; but it is not a

good treatment for someone with widespread or continually active psoriasis.

Chapter 7

1. A variety of vitamins and minerals encourage the healthy growth of hair and nails. Oils can be massaged into the scalp keeping it free of irritation for prolonged periods.

2. PsoriNail™, Onyplex™ and other products can be used to harden nails so they don't break as easily.

Chapter 8

1. Suggestions are given for clothing and fabrics that irritate your skin the least. Knowledge of clothing types and the materials they are made of can determine how irritation-free you will be and the amount of damage that can be caused by the products you put on your skin.

2. Special tan-through swimsuits are offered by at least two companies (see appendix). The fabric(s) allows access to the sun without your skin actually being visible to others.

3. Pant liners and thermal underwear and undershirts can be used to protect your clothes from staining by medications or oils which you apply to your skin.

Chapter 9

1. The value of an active life cannot be understated. The healthier you are the better your body can deal with any disorder. Activities should be chosen that are pleasurable and varied to maintain your interest and to achieve a balanced usage of all parts. The activity should be easy to incorporate into your daily schedule to ensure you don't become a "drop-out."

2. Taking your pulse allows you to instantly read your exertion level and overall condition. Your pulse reflects your physical and even your emotional condition. Your pulse may easily be taken at your wrist or neck.

Chapter 10

1. The skin is the largest organ of the body. It controls water loss and moisture level and when out of balance can become dry causing irritation, pain and inflammation. Moisturizing agents, which prevent moisture evaporation while not reducing the ability of the skin to breathe adequately, are the most desirable for preventing dryness.

2. A description of bodily organs related to the digestive and eliminative systems is presented. Improper functioning of the colon is considered by many doctors to be the origin of many diseases, including psoriasis. Optimizing the colon's ability to function is important. Understanding the interaction of your organs will help you notice the signals that indicate possible malfunction.

3. The T-cells and their importance to psoriasis research.

Chapter 11

1. The acupuncturist looks at the whole system. They get a picture of both the physical and the non-physical. Insights are drawn on whether all bodily functions are operating optimally.

2. Dr. Fred Siciliano comments on acupuncture. The goal of acupuncture is to assist the body to function at its optimum, facilitating self-healing. Dr. Siciliano answers the questions: How does acupuncture work?

3. Dr. John Pagano comments on chiropractic. His book and his articles focus on spinal health and nutrition. Dr. Pagano states that throughout the Edgar Cayce readings, maintaining the integrity of the human spine by manual manipulation rings loud and clear as a major health measure. There is a direct connection between correct spinal alignment and the health of your internal organs. The doctor doesn't heal anything; he removes blockages to allow the body to heal itself.

4. Dr. Karl V. Holmquist comments on chiropractic. His self-help book, Home Chiropractic Handbook, was written to help people in the process of becoming healthy; he does not intend the book to replace doctors or chiropractors.

5. Dr. Velma Scott comments that a flexible spine, nutrition and a happy positive attitude is the road to good health.

6. Yoga is one activity which will keep the spine fluid and flexible. A fluid spine accompanied with good posture has been hailed for centuries in many Far East countries as a necessity for good health.

Chapter 12

1. The Canadian Psoriasis Foundation (C.P.F.) comments on a Swedish preparation, "Psori-Aid" capsules, now called "X-ORI," in which the natural active ingredient is easily metabolized, symptoms decrease and cell function returns to normal. Sold in Canada and the United States.

2. Dr. Karl V. Holmquist points out that every drug that is either swallowed by mouth or injected by needle is absorbed into the bloodstream and pumped to every organ, all tissue and ultimately to every cell of the body.

Chapter 13

1. Gerovital H3 (GH3) was developed in 1956 for the treatment of degenerative diseases and revitalizing action in advanced age. It is administered orally and by injection.

2. Once in the body, GH3 breaks down into two constituents which stimulate the good intestinal flora and participate in the making of other vital substances.

3. The tissue regenerating action of Gerovital H3 is evident especially on the skin and extraskeleton where it produces a rejuvenating appearance.

Chapter 14

1. An article published by the National Psoriasis Foundation discusses a particular dietary means of slowing cell turnover to combat the too-rapid growth of skin cells that cause psoriasis - starvation. Of course, this "cure" is worse than the disease.

2. Some general principles for maintaining good health include regulating the types of food consumed, the amount consumed, and the combination

of foods consumed at one sitting. Psoriasis patients should refrain from food groups that are not healthy, such as "junk food," so as to minimize reactions such as severe itching. However, total exclusion of this type of food is not necessary for all, as long as moderation is practiced.

3. Writer Jackman Gillette observed that we consume more protein than our bodies need. He concluded that protein starvation will ultimately result in the stoppage of the scaling process and a clearing of psoriatic lesion. However, this no-protein diet does have damaging side effects and extended programs could cause starvation.

4. Dr. Kenneth Thane Walker describes the essence of good eating habits, "Everything in moderation, including moderation."

5. The best diet: don't eat the same thing twice in one week; eat fiber; eat less; drink water often every day.

Chapter 15

1. Dr. Michael Holick says patients had a good to excellent response to vitamin D therapy.

2. Our environment is full of stressful chemicals, such as food additives and pesticides, that need to be processed by the liver so that they can be eliminated by the body. Christopher Hobbs states that medicinal herbs are still used by the majority of the population in the world today for prevention of disease and restoration of wellness. Milk Thistle is a powerful herb that helps restore the liver's health.

3. Dr. Daniel Mowrey states that psoriasis is related to endotoxin concentrations (poison contained in the cell walls of some bacteria), and the production of harmful leukotriene cells (radical oxygen molecules that interfere with normal liver function). Milk Thistle treatment slows down the development of these harmful leukotriene cells.

4. Various herbal and vitamin remedies and sources are noted. Two important notes: vitamin supplements can be dangerous when taken at high levels; vitamins/minerals should be gained in the food we eat and not through artificial supplements which should only by used as a last resort.

5. Acidophilus is a source of friendly intestinal bacteria and acidophilus aids the intestines and colon in working at their optimum condition - clean.

6. Dr. William Lane's research showed shark cartilage contains a natural occurring compound known to fight inflammation such as that which occurs in psoriasis. A recommended commercial form of shark cartilage.

Chapter 16

1. Dr. Allan Cott comments on benefits of fasting. Fasting is considered the ultimate diet. He clarifies fasting as a health benefit not to be confused with starving. The body does not consume itself in any vital way even during an extended fast. People who have fasted usually discover new reservoirs of strength and vitality.

2. Dr. Roy Walford comments on his research on caloric-restrictions which should allow a healthier and longer life.

Chapter 17

1. When colon elimination is hindered, toxins are reabsorbed into the bloodstream, lowering the body's defenses against bacteria and viruses. The colon is a natural sewage reservoir and is the most abused organ of the entire body.

2. Colonic therapy can remove the years of buildup within the colon. Colonics are designed to tune up the system so it becomes more capable of healing itself.

3. Good colon health habits: cultivate bowel movements at the same time, two to three times a day. Drink plenty of water and take acidophilus.

4. The Welles Step puts a person into the natural position of squatting thus eliminating the undue strain applied to the abdominal wall and bowel by the modern toilet.

5. Internal cleansing programs using natural substances such as psyllium are recommended to complement colonics.

Chapter 18

1. Louise Hay in her book, "You Can Heal Your Life", comments on a path to improved health. Psoriasis' probable cause is fear of being hurt, deadening the senses and the self, and refusing to accept responsibility for our own feelings.

2. Neuro-Linguistic Programming (NLP) you create your own future.

3. Dick Sutphen comments on accessing altered states of consciousness to improve your health. Sutphen gives an example of a woman who never allowed her true self to be exposed to others for fear of rejection. After acknowledging the fear she began revealing herself to others, and her skin condition cleared up entirely.

4. An evolutionary attitude results in the opening of many doors.

Chapter 19

1. Imagery and its value. Imagery is a clear sequence of mental pictures of what you want starting from where you are, and ending at where you want to be. The conscious repetition of these pictures will produce the desired results.

Chapter 20

1. Dr. John Harrison in his book, "Love Your Disease", comments that all illness is a consequence of stress from a childhood survival adaptation. Stress is self-created, and a synonym for fear.

2. Louise Hay in her book, "You Can Heal Your Life", comments that to release the past, we must be willing to forgive. We need to choose to release the past and forgive everyone, ourselves included.

3. N.L.P. Comprehensive teaches that forgiveness is not for that other person or the world but for you. You learn to forgive yourself then you learn to forgive others.

4. With David Harp's forgiveness meditation you forgive the person, not their behavior. Letting go of anger and of feelings of having been wronged is a very freeing experience.

Elliott Douglas Derzaph

Appendices

Elliott Douglas Derzaph

Glossary

acidophilus - a source of friendly intestinal bacteria
APC - (Antigen-presenting cell) cells that grasp things that appear foreign and trigger an immune system response.
attribute - a quality or characteristic.
autoimmune - our immune system attacks normal cells usually when the body overproduces a substance in the body.
bioavailability - the degree of medication that becomes available to the body.
biologics - a class of drugs which inhibit highly specific parts like the immune system processes that lead to psoriasis diseases.
calcitriol - Vitamin "D3" in the kidney, whose main function is to increase absorption from the intestine.
calcipotriol/calcipotriene - generic names of the topical drug vitamin D3 analog, used for people with mild to moderate psoriasis. As effective as a midpotency topical steroid without the side effects. It doesn't thin out the skin, and it doesn't cause a rebound of psoriasis. Available by prescription as Dovonex.
CD4 - is a T cell or helper cell.
chiropractic - a therapeutic system based upon the premise that disease is caused by interference with nerve function, and that normal condition can be restored by adjusting the segments of the spinal column.
Clinical trial - have a set of rules for safety and the product's effectiveness to do the research determining if new treatments or drugs should be pursued. Usually occur when products available do not solve the problem. Unknown side effects. Always, do your homework and ask any question you or your doctor recommends before entering into the trial.
Corticosteroids - secretion by the adrenal gland made up of cortisone-like molecules. Also produced synthetically for use as a drug with diseases including inflammatory conditions and is associated with many side-effects including emotional changes, ulcers and increased susceptibility to infection.
Cyclosporine - a drug used for severe psoriasis that suppresses the immune system.
cysteine - a component of nearly all proteins, obtained by the reduction of cystine.

cystine - an amino acid occurring in most proteins, especially the keratins in hair.

detoxify - to rid of poison or the effect of poison.

DNA (deoxyribonucleic acid) - found chiefly in the nucleus of cells, whose function is to transfer genetic characteristics, and in the synthesis of protein. New DNA research, encouraged and funded by the N.P.F., will quite probably create a cure for psoriasis. But due to necessary research cost and legal and medical requirements, it will probably be another few years before psoriasis sufferers will benefit.

Dovonex - the brand name for topical D3. Effective for short term clearing of psoriasis. Dovonex slows cell division, causes normal cell differentiation, and regulates immune function in the skin.

endorphins - any of several naturally occurring chemicals (proteins) in the brain, involved in reducing or eliminating pain and in enhancing pleasure. Studies show that acupuncture may induce the production of endorphins.

etretinate (Tegison) - a potent oral drug effective for pustular and erythrodermic psoriasis is being replaced by a new drug called "acitretin." Drinking alcohol while taking this drug may cause birth defects.

fiber - the wholly or partially indigestible parts of the plants that stimulate contractions in the intestine; bulk or roughage. Note: all fiber is not the same and different types of fiber perform different functions.

follicle - a small cavity, sac or gland enclosing a hair and from which hair grows.

folliculitis - hair follicles inflamed.

fusion protein molecule - (now known as IL-2 Fusion Protein) a product being researched using genetic engineering to bind with activated T-cells and destroy them leaving normal cells alone. Research demonstrated that psoriasis is an immune-mediated disorder.

gene - the unit of heredity transmitted in the chromosome and that, partially through interaction with other genes, controls the development of hereditary characteristics; 200 genes are in the area that are considered to hold the blueprint for Psoriasis with 11 single genetic mutations identified at this time.

hereditary - passing or capable of passing, naturally from parents to offspring.

healing - growing sound, getting well, regaining health.

heredity - the transmission of genetic characters from parents to offspring, variations resulting from the interaction of the genes and the environment.
hydration - to combine chemically with water in its molecular form.
hydroxyurea - a drug that inhibits cells with rapid growth.
hyperplasia - rapid skin cell growth.
hyperproliferation - over production of skin cells
imagery - the formation of mental images and/or collective images especially those produced by the use of imagination. Specific thoughts of many sequential images flowing in a specific direction.
inverse/flexural psoriasis - a type of psoriasis found in areas where the skin folds or flexes.
keratinocyte - psoriasis lesions are considered to develop because of the accelerated growth of this type of skin cells.
linguistic - the science of meaningful units of language.
loma psoriasis - a natural homeopathic oral medication based on a mineral therapy research.
metabolic - affected by metabolism, undergoing change.
methotrexate (MTX) - medication used to slow cell production and decrease inflammation.
mucus - a lubricating secretion used mainly to aid the transport and the breakdown of foods.
neuro - indicating an association with the nervous system.
neuron - a nerve cell with its processes, constituting the structural and functional unit of nerve tissue.
nervous system - a network of cells to conduct information in running the whole body.
occlusive - a blockage or closing of a passageway in the body.
parapsoriasis - a group of skin conditions that are not related to psoriasis. Psoriasis is not parapsoriasis and does not turn into parapsoriasis.
pathology - the study of disease, its causes and effects, especially the effects of disease on body tissue.
procedure - the act or manner of a surgical operation.
psychosomatic - noting a physical disorder that is caused by, or notably influenced by, the emotional state of the patient.
roughage - food containing a high proportion of indigestible cellulose which stimulates contractions in the intestines. Useful in the digestive process to move food along at a healthy pace while assisting in the maintenance of the intestine. (Also see "fiber.")

salicylic acid - a product used on the scales causing the skin to swell, soften and detach; scale lifters; tar products are an alternative
soma - the body.
somatic temperature variance - example - psoriasis - the irritated area of the skin becomes hotter than the non-irritated/normal skin of the body. The increased production of cells raises the normal temperature of the skin, which normally causes itching.
steroid - skin cell growth is slowed down where steroid medication is applied, decreases inflammation; can be compounded with salicylic acid.
stress - causes our skin to loose its ability to hold water.
substance P - a neuropeptide released by sensory fibers in the skin.
superantigens - proteins are made up of microbes including bacterium or viruses that stimulate the immune system to have an abnormally strong reaction.
superpotent - the strongest class of corticosteroids.
synapse - the tiny gap between two neurons or between a neuron and a muscle across which nerve impulses are transmitted through the action of neurotransmitters. When an impulse reaches the end of one neuron it causes the release of a neurotransmitter that diffuses across the gap to trigger an impulse in the other neuron or muscle.
Tachyphylaxis - when medications stop being effective (seen most often with topical steroids). The phenomenon of losing effectiveness appears to happen with many Psoriasis products.
T cells - a type of white blood cell that release cytokines (chemicals used by the immune system to communicate messages). Cytokines, in people with psoriasis, tell our skins cells to reproduce too rapidly (10 times as fast as healthy skin) which activate T cells in a cycle that keeps forming new skin creating lesions. T cells are the main component of our lymphatic system. (Helper T cells - immune response) (Killer T cells - destroy perceived foreign cells)
TNF-alpha (tumor necrosis factor-alpha) - promotes inflammation to fight infections; a protein that helps regulate the body's immune response; overproduced by people with psoriasis in joints and skins
visualization - to make perceptible to the mind or imagination, to recall or form mental images or pictures. Usually thought of as a snapshot of one or a few images, whereas imagery is a more

creative and less restrictive picture of a reality you wish to create. Many people use visualization to picture a specific goal. Whereas imagery creates a flow of pictures taking you from your present reality to the outcome of your goals. Visualization creates the individual and specific pictures of your new reality while imagery puts them together in a chain significant to your desired direction and outcome. (Also see "imagery.")

Forms of Psoriasis

Annularis - Psoriasis in ring-shaped patches
Arthropathica - A form associated with chronic arthritis
Buccalis - Marked by white, thickened patches in mucous membranes of cheeks, gums, tongue
Circinata - (see Annularis)
Diffusa - Coalescence of large contiguous lesions (Bakers, grocers, bricklayers itch, etc.)
Discoides - Occurring in solid patches
Figurata - Lesions in curved linear patterns
Follicularis - Small, scaly lesions located at openings of sebaceous and sweat glands
Guttata - Occurs in small, distinct, irregular patches
Gyrata - Having serpentine arrangement
Inveterata - With confluent lesions and thickening and hardening skin
Linguae - (See Buccalis above)
Nummularis - In circular patches that resembles coins
Osteacea - In Old, thick, tough patches covered with scales resembling outside of oyster shells
Palmaris et plantaris - Syphiloderm of palms or soles
Punctata - Lesions consist of minute, red, pinhead-shaped papules, often surmounted with pearly scales
Pustular p. - Lesions are covered with pustules
Rupioides - Rupia-like crusts (skin eruptions usually from syphilis)
Universalis - Lesions over whole body

Types of Psoriasis

Annular psoriasis - red ring shaped; scaly pustular; shed; lasts months to years; mild.

Acropustulosis psoriasis (acrodermatitis continua of Hallopeau) - extremely rare; lesions on ends of toes and fingers.

Erythrodermic psoriasis - 4% of patients; rarest; reddening and shedding; severe itching and pain; affects most of the body; can cause death; can cause substantial protein and fluid loss.

Exanthematic psoriasis - often triggered by infection; pustules; normally clears when infection clears.

Generalized pustular psoriasis (von Zumbusch type) - reddened skin on wide areas of skin which is tender and painful; can be triggered by infection, withdrawal of steroids and some beta-blockers; can be life threatening; and can often require hospitalization.

Guttate psoriasis - 18% of patients and 2nd most common type; triggers include infections, stress, injury, respiratory (upper) infections and some drugs; lesions smaller, thinner and less scaling.

Inverse psoriasis - 10% of patients; found in skin folds; smooth, large, very red and lack scales.

Localized pustular psoriasis (palmo-plantar pustulosis) - affects palms and soles; triggered by stress and infection; stubborn and can be disabling.

Plaque psoriasis (psoriasis vulgaris) - most common type; elevated; thick; usually red and dot shaped to begin with; silvery white in appearance later; infects small to very large size area; plaques can merge; triggers include stress, injury, irritation, and others.

Pustular psoriasis - 5% of patients; rare; cyclical; can react to internal and external medications, systemic steroids, infection and stress; usually appears as small blisters then forms pustules and scales off.

Optimum Schedule & Curriculum

DAILY

- Drink a glass of water every 2 hours you are awake
- Take a shower or bath
- Bathe/swim/steam every day if possible, when highly irritated
- Follow shower or bath by lubricating skin with lotion or oil
- Take one capsule of acidophilus
- Eat fresh fruits and vegetables
- Exercise 15 minutes each and every day at a minimum
- Cultivate 1 to 3 bowel movements a day
- Affirm goals
- Visualize a healthy psoriasis-free body five minutes before going to sleep

WEEKLY

- Bathe/swim/steam for 30 minutes at least once a week
- Outdoor activity/sunshine for 60 minutes at a minimum (preferably not all at one time)
- Juice or water, only, one full day a week

MONTHLY

- Massage for 30 minutes

SIX MONTHS

- Colonics (3 times in one week) regular maintenance
- Colonics (as often as needed when your system needs help)

YEARLY

- Contribute to Ontological and Emotional Intelligence research, the National Psoriasis Foundation and the Canadian Psoriasis Foundation

LIFE

- Practice emotional maintenance
- Read all information available on psoriasis
- Use natural products including natural drugs (herbs/homeopathic)
- Consume the minimum amount of sugar, caffeine, alcohol, fat, meats and dairy products
- In emergencies or critical situations be sensible
- Always seek out the best help you can find
- Keep abreast of the overall healthy habits of our society
- Maintain open communication with health practitioners
- Visualize a healthy body inside and out
- Appreciate life and laugh often
- Keep your spine fluid with activity such as yoga
- Keep your mind open and thinking
- Nurture your self-concept and self-worth
- Seek studies in Ontology and Emotional Intelligence

Always be conscious of your activities and use your health practitioners to guide you. Maintain an exchange of knowledge with your practitioner. Keep in mind you have your body for life.

EDUCATION IS THE ANSWER

PLEASE SHARE YOUR KNOWLEDGE

SHARE PUBLICATIONS OR INFORMATION WITH FRIENDS, RELATIVES, AND ACQUAINTANCES

Elliott Douglas Derzaph

Psoriasis Information Resources and Organizations throughout The World

UNITED STATES

The National Psoriasis Foundation (NPF/USA)

The two organizations that have been the most helpful, over the years in researching psoriasis have been the Public Library and the National Psoriasis Foundation. A portion of the information presented in this book came directly from the Foundation's printed material for members.

The NPF/USA offers booklets and a bimonthly bulletin on a variety of related subject matter. Membership fees are by contribution - which may be nominal or as much as you wish. The organization is non-profit, allowing tax deductible contributions to a worthwhile cause.

The NPF/USA sponsors local psoriasis communication networks so that people with psoriasis have the chance to interact. Networks give people the opportunity to attend educational meetings, participate in self-help activities and initiate community awareness about their disorder. They offer an educational opportunity to understand and cope with psoriasis.

(This program and information is continually being updated by the NPF/USA. I suggest that you contact them directly for the most up-to-date details on any of their services. NPF/USA will always do its best to assist anyone in fulfilling their needs.)

An application for membership in NPF can be found at the end of this book.

National Psoriasis Foundation, 6600 SW 92nd Ave., Suite 300, Portland, OR 97223 (503) 244-7404 or (800) 723-9166

Dermatology Center, U.C.L.A. Medical Plaza, Ste. 465, 200 U.C.L.A. Medical Plaza, Los Angeles, CA 90024

University of California-Irvine, College of Medicine, Dept. of Dermatology, Irvine, CA 92717

University of California, School of Medicine, San Francisco, Dept. of Dermatology, San Francisco, CA 94143

Stanford University School of Medicine, Dept. of Dermatology, Stanford, CA 94305

Psoriasis Research Institute, P.O. Box V, Palo Alto, CA 94305

Southern California Dermatology and Psoriasis Center, Santa Monica, California 90404

Columbia University College of Physicians & Surgeons, Dept. of Dermatology, N.Y., N.Y. 10032

Duke University Medical Center, Dept. of Dermatology, Durham, NC 27710

Harvard Medical School, Dept. of Dermatology, Boston, MA 02114

University of Miami, School of Medicine, Dept. of Dermatology, Miami, FL 33101

University of Michigan Medical School, Dept. of Dermatology, Ann Arbor, MI 48109

New England Journal of Medicine (NEJM), 1440 Main St., Waltham, MA 02154-1649

University of Pennsylvania, School of Medicine, Dept. of Dermatology, Philadelphia, PA 19104

Temple University, School of Medicine, Dept. of Dermatology, Philadelphia, PA 19140

University of Utah, College of Medicine, Dermatology, Salt Lake City, UT 84132

Washington Hospital Center, Washington, D.C. 20010

Yale University, Dept. of Dermatology, New Haven, CT 06510

The Edgar Cayce Foundation, Medical Research Division, P.O. Box 595, Virginia Beach, VA., 23451 (or) Association for Research and Enlightenment, 215 67th St., Virginia Beach, VA 23451

American Academy of Dermatology, 1567 Maple Ave., Evanston, IL 60204 (offers general knowledge booklets on skin problems at a small cost)

American Medical Association, AMA Publications, 515 N. State, Chicago, IL 60610 (Offers a variety of general knowledge booklets specifically on skin diseases, for a small charge.)

American Academy of Dermatology, 930 N. Meacham Rd., P.O. Box 4014, Schaumburg, IL 60168

National Health Information Clearing House, P.O. Box 1133, Washington, D.C. 20013

National Institute of Skin Disease, Information Clearing House, Box AMS, 9000 Rockville Pike, Bethesda, MD 20892

OTHER ENGLISH SPEAKING COUNTRIES

Canada
Psoriasis Society of Canada, PO Box 25015, Halifax, NS, B3M 4H4, Tel: (902) 443-8680 or (800) 656-4434

Australia
Psoriasis Association of Victoria, P.O. Box 1151, Glen Waverly, Victoria 3150 Tel: 61-03-9813-8080

United Kingdom
Psoriasis Arthropathy Alliance, P.O. Box 111, St. Albans, Hertfordshire AL2 3JQ Tel: 011-44-1-923-672-837

NON-ENGLISH SPEAKING COUNTRIES

Belgium
Vlaamse Vereniging van Psoriasis Patineten, V.V.P.P., Beervelde-Dorp, 39, 9080 Lochristi

China
China Psoriasis Foundation, Dept. of Dermatology, Air Force General Hospital, PLA, 30 Fucheng Road, Beijing 100036

Denmark
Danmarks Psoriasis Forening, Kloverprisvej 10 B, 2650 Hvidovre

Estonia
Eesti Psoriaasi Liit EPsol, Komeedi 13-4, 10122 Tallinn

France
Association Pour La Lutte Contre Le Psoriasis, 1 allec du Stade, 95610 Eragny

Germany
Duetscher Psoriasis Bund e.v., Oberaltenalle 20A, 22081 Hamburg 76

Iceland
SPOEX, Bolholt 6,105 Reykjavik

Israel
Israel Psoriasis Association, P.O. Box 13275, Tel-Aviv

Italy
A.S.N.P.V., Via Bergognone 43, 20144 Milan

A.DI.PSO, Via Tacito, 90, 00193 Roma

Lithuania
Psoriasis Society of Lithuania, K. Petrausko g. 26, 3000 Kaunas, p.k. 2095

Norway
Norsk Psoriasisforbund, Pb 6547, Etterstad, 0606 Oslo

Spain
ACCIO Psoriasi, Avgda. De Vallvidera, 73, 08017 Barcelona

Sweden
Svanska Psoriasisforbundet, Rokerigatan 19, S-121 92 Johanneshov

Switzerland
SPVG, Postfach 8048, Zurich

References & Product Resources

Books (United States)

Healing Psoriasis, by Dr. John Pagano, 1991, 346 pp. (Voted "Best Health Book of the Year" by the North American Bookdealers Exchange.) The Pagano Organization, Inc.

Psoriasis: A Guide to One of the Commonest Skin Diseases, by Dr. Ronald A. Marks, 1981, 107 pp. Arco Publishing, Inc.

Psoriasis: The Story of a Man who Helped Himself, by Jackman Gillette, 1980, 100 pp. Horizon Press, New York.

Managing Your Psoriasis, by Dr. Nicholas J. Lowe, 1993, 115 pp. Mastermedia Limited. (This book explains medical approaches, medication and types of psoriasis. The author has set up psoriasis treatment centers.)

Andrews' Diseases of the Skin, by George Clinton Andrews, 1982. 1108 pp. Philadelphia, $106.00

The Ancient Art of Self Healing, by Yogi Bhajan, 1982. 150 pp. West Anandpur.

Colon Health: the Key to a Vibrant Life, by Norman W. Walker D.Sc., Ph.D., 1979. 131 pp. Norwalk Press.

The Colon Health Handbook, by Robert Gray, 1986. 77 pp. Emerald Publishing.

Composition of Foods, by the U.S. Government, Agriculture Handbook #8, Consumer and Food Economics Institute, Agricultural Research Service, U.S. Dept. of Agriculture, Superintendent of Documents, U.S. Government Printing Office, Washington, D.C., 20402

Elliott Douglas Derzaph

The Edgar Cayce Handbook for Health through Drugless Therapy, by Dr. Harold J. Reilly and Ruth Hagy Brod, 1975. 495 pp. Berkley Publishing.

The Emotional Hostage, by Leslie Cameron-Bandler & Michael Lebeau, 1986. 220 pp. Real People Press.

Gerovital H3, by the National Institute of Gerontology and Geriatrics, 1982. 96 pp. Phoenix Creation Ltd., Vancouver, B.C.

Gray's Anatomy, by Henry Gray, F.R.S., 1977. 1257 pp. Gramercy Books.

Healing Visualizations - Creating Health through Imagery, by Gerald Epstein, M.D., 1989. 226 pp. Bantam Books.

How Juices Restore Health Naturally by Salem Kirban, 1981. 107 pp. Salem Kirban, Inc.

The Incredible Machine, by National Geographical Society, 1986. 384 pp.

The Incredible Credible Cosmic Consciousness Diet, by Harvey Cohen, Ph. D. Psycho-Dynamics.

Lick the Sugar Habit, by Nancy Appleton, Ph.D, 1985. 162 pp. Warner Books.

Love Your Disease, by John Harrison, M.D., 1984. 388 pp. Hay House, Inc.

Medical Dictionary for the Non-Professional, by Charles F. Chapman, 1984. 440 pp. Barron's Educational Series.

Nontoxic and Natural, by Debra Lynn Dadd, 1984. 289 pp. Jeremy P. Tarcher, Inc.

Survival into the 21st Century, by Viktoras Kulvinskas, M.S., 1975. 312 pp. 21st Century Publications.

Tissue Cleansing through Bowel Management, by Bernard Jensen D.C., 1981. 171 pp. (Published by Bernard Jensen)

Total Fitness: in 30 minutes a week, by Dr. Laurende B. Morehouse and Leonard Gross, 1975. 255 pp. Simon & Schuster, Inc.

What Your Doctor Won't Tell You, by Jane Heimlich, 1990. 288 pp. HarperCollins.

Your Body is your Best Doctor, by Melvin E. Page, D.D.S. and H. Leon Abrams, Jr., 1972. 236 pp. Keats Publishing, Inc.

Your Gut Feelings, by Dr. Henry D. Janowitz, 1987. 204 pp. Consumers Union, Yonkers, N.Y.

Books (United Kingdom)

Psoriasis: A Practical Guide to Coping, by Dr. Caroline Wilson, 1989. 96 pp. The Crowood Press, Ramsbury, Marlborough, Wiltshire SNS 2HE (this book is part of the Crowood Health Guides Series) (In the U.S. - Trafalgar Square, P.O. Box 257, Howe Hill Rd., North Pomfret, VT 05053)

Additional Resources

Sources of Cosmetic (cosmeceutical) Cover-Up products.

       Dermablend Corrective Cosmetics 877-900-6700
       Faye Mendelsohn Cosmetics 800-500-3293
       Kryolan 800-579-6526
       Lydia O'Leary Cosmetics/Covermark 800-524-1120
       Max Factor (check your drug store)
       Curad Scar Therapy Cosmetic Pads 800-227-4703

Video - "Psoriasis: Treatments for Today, Research for Tomorrow" over seven hours of up-to-date information from the 30th Psoriasis Conference. Call the National Psoriasis Foundation (503) 244-7404 or (800) 723-9166

Writers with Psoriasis who wrote books about characters with Psoriasis: John Updike in the book "The Centaur" and Dennis Potter in the book "Hide and Seek."

Elliott Douglas Derzaph

The Edgar Cayce Foundation, Medical Research Division, P.O. Box 595, Virginia Beach, VA, 23451 (or) Association for Research and Enlightenment (A.R.E.), 215 67th St., Virginia Bch., VA 23451

Solar type swimwear:
Coolware Co. Inc., 5801 Coyote Pass, Shingle Springs, CA 95682 (specify what type of clothing you are seeking) 800-235-3003
Lifestyles Direct, P.O. Box 152929, Tampa, FL 33684 (800) 951-2001

The Welles Step, Welles Enterprises, 6565 Balbow Ave., San Diego, CA 92111 (619) 473-8011

The American Association of Acupuncture and Oriental Medicine, Raleigh, N.C. (919) 787-5181

Vitamin Books and Products

The Vitamin Bible, by Earl Mindell, Warner Books.

Note: Ask your local nutritionist to suggest quality distributors of vitamins.

Prescription Drug Books and Products

The AMA Guide to Prescription and Non-Prescription (Over-the-Counter) Drugs, Random House.

The Essential Guide to Prescription Drugs, by James W. Long, Harper and Row.

Pharmacy Service Prescription Drug Handbook, A.A.R.P. Pharmacy Service, 1 Prince St., Alexandria, VA 22314

The Pill Book Guide to Safe Drug Use, by Harold M. Silverman, Pharm. D., Bantam Books.

The mail order pharmacies offer low prices on psoriasis, specific, prescription and non-prescription drugs. They normally deliver in about one week. However, watch the super discount drugstore chains, sometimes they offer products at very competitive prices. Always compare prices before making any purchase.

Elliott Douglas Derzaph

Home Therapy Lighting

Listed below are a few companies that offer units designed specifically for psoriasis home therapy:

    American Sunlight, Inc.
    7266-D Edinger Ave.
    Huntington Beach, CA 92647
    (714) 375-7900

    Daavlin
    205 West Bement St.
    P.O. Box 626
    Bryan, OH 43506
    (800) 322-8546 (USA)
    (419) 636-6304

    National Biological Corp.
    1532 Enterprise Parkway
    Twinsburg, OH 44087
    (800) 338-5045
    (330) 425-3535

    Ultralite Enterprises, Inc.
    390 Farmer Ct.
    Lawrenceville (Atlanta), GA 30245
    (800) 241-7506
    (770) 963-0594

    Solarc Systems Inc.
    12 Parker Court
    Barrie, ON, Canada L4N 2A6
    (866) 813-3357
    (705) 739-8279

Laser Resources

Candela Corporation - 508-358-7637
Cynosure - 800-866-2966
PhotoMedex - 877-449-8722

Elliott Douglas Derzaph

Information and Applications

Readers may wish to join a psoriasis association in their country. A list of all such associations known to the author, is provided in the Appendix, in the section: Psoriasis Information Resources.

National Psoriasis Foundation (NPF)

To make it easier for the millions of American and Canadian sufferers to join their respective associations, we have printed application forms for both. Simply copy the form, complete it, and mail it to the address provided. National psoriasis associations provide general information about psoriasis, other educational material, and a description of their programs in its initial free packet, prior to joining. After joining, you will be sent information about the associations' programs and additional educational material.

Psoriasis Society of Canada

The information offered by the Canadian association tends to complement, rather than duplicate, what is offered by the NPF; so the author suggests that readers join both associations to evaluate the type and degree of assistance offered by each. After one year, you can choose to renew one, or both, based on the help you have received.

Psoriasis: The Struggle and the Triumph
A Healthy Transformation for Everyone Living with Psoriasis

National Psoriasis Foundation (NPF)

(COPY THIS FORM AND MAIL)

National Psoriasis Foundation
6600 SW 92nd Avenue, Ste. 300
Portland, OR 97223-7195
Tel: 503-244-7404
Tel: 800-723-9166
Fax: 503-245-0626

www.psoriasis.org

Yes, please send me a FREE packet of information about psoriasis, along with information on how to join NPF.

or

My donation is enclosed. Please start my NPF membership subscriptions, in addition to sending me a free information packet.

My Name _____

Address _____

City State Zip _____

Referring Physician or Medical Facility (optional)_____

_____

Elliott Douglas Derzaph

Psoriasis: The Struggle and the Triumph
A Healthy Transformation for Everyone Living with Psoriasis

Psoriasis Society of Canada (National Office)

(COPY THIS FORM AND MAIL)

Psoriasis Society of Canada
PO Box 25015, Halifax, NS
B3M 4H4, Canada
Tel: (902) 443-8680
Tel: (800) 656-4494
Fax: (902) 443-2073

www.PsoriasisSociety.org

Membership
Donation

Yes, I want to become a member of the Society. (Please call for current membership rates.) Please put me on your mailing list to receive the National Psoriasis Newsletter.

Yes, I would like to donate $_____ to the Society to support research, conferences, workshops and promote awareness of psoriasis.

Name _____

Address _____

City _____

Postal Code/Prov. _____

Telephone _____

Elliott Douglas Derzaph

"Psoriasis: The Struggle and The Triumph"
Contact Information

(COPY THIS FORM AND MAIL)

Psoriasis Advisor, P.O. Box 643038, West Los Angeles, CA 90064-3038

www.PsoriasisAdvisor.com   email: Info@PsoriasisAdvisor.com

Yes, I want to share the following information with the Psoriasis Advisor who will disseminate the edited information to people with Psoriasis.

_____

_____

_____

_____

_____

_____

_____

_____

Name _____

Address _____

City _____

State or Postal / Zip or Postal Code _____

_____Yes, please put me on your mailing list to receive future Psoriasis updates.

Elliott Douglas Derzaph

Psoriasis: The Struggle and the Triumph
A Healthy Transformation for Everyone Living with Psoriasis

"*Psoriasis: The Struggle and The Triumph*" Order Form

(COPY THIS FORM AND MAIL)

Use this form to order "*Psoriasis: The Struggle and The Triumph*", if you cannot find it at your usual source of self help books or do not have access to the web site.

Libraries: Please contact publisher for library pricing.
Resellers: Please contact publisher for resale pricing.

_____ *Psoriasis: The Struggle and The Triumph* x **$12.95** = _____
Quantity   Cost   Amount

                       Postage and Handling*: $_____
                       6% Sales Tax: (IN only) $_____
                       Total Enclosed: ($US) $_____

* U.S.A. Only: Postage and Handling - $5.75 for the first book and $1.00 for each additional book.

MAIL BOOKS TO:
Name: _____
Address _____
City: _____ State: _____ Zip/Postal Code: _____

MAIL ORDERS TO PUBLISHER:
    1stBooks Library
    1663 Liberty Drive, Ste. 200
    Bloomington, IN 47403 USA

PUBLISHER CONTACT INFO.:
    www.1stbooks.com (web page)
    Info@1stbooks.com (email)
    888-839-8640 (Toll-free)
    812-339-6000 (Outside USA & Canada)
    812-339-6554 (Fax)

Elliott Douglas Derzaph

A Poem

__SUN WARMED PEOPLE__

From sun to sea…
I dream to live…
From rough to smooth…
From red to pink…
From hot to warm…
From dry to moist…
From distant to close…
From a frown to a smile…
From anger to understanding…
From unknown to known…
From whispers to conversations…
From acquaintances to friends…
From a touch to a hug…
From fear to love…
To finally seeing me.

About the Author

Elliott Douglas Derzaph was born and raised in Canada. After high school, he traveled and lived in various cities in Central and Western Canada. In the mid 1970's, he immigrated to the United States where he became an American citizen. He lived in Hawaii for 5 years while attending school studying Ontology in which he later obtained a degree. During the same period, he was the personal aide to writer, psychoanalyst and public speaker, Dr. Kenneth (Thane) Walker.

Upon leaving Hawaii and settling in Los Angeles, he entered the world of computers, later specializing in Project Management. In 1990, the Author started his own business as a Project Manager including Research & Development and Consulting.

Elliott has discovered the necessity of life-long learning and is always pursuing further education. Elliott has been studying his avocation, the field of Emotional Intelligence since 1974. Elliott is considered an idea-man who always follows through. Elliott is an entrepreneur who has been in business mainly as a sole proprietor. Elliott has written books, scripts and poems as well as doing volunteer work since his youth, including marketing, text compilation (including a book on Ontology), video and digitizing. Elliott regularly contributes to a variety of non-profit organizations and has won "Man of the Year" twice for his volunteer work. He has traveled throughout North and Central America as well as Europe. He has a loving wife and son.

The author was prompted to write this book by the questions of his many friends, acquaintances and family, who were curious about the psoriasis data he had started to compile since 1978. Further impetus was given by his conversations with many psoriasis sufferers who indicated there was an extreme lack of information on the subject.

The author felt that if just one idea was helpful to each reader in relieving some of the discomfort of psoriasis, it was well worth his efforts in writing this book.

Printed in the United Kingdom
by Lightning Source UK Ltd.
105194UKS00001B/162